THE SMART GUIDE TO

D1509440

Managing Stress

BY B

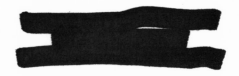

The Smart Guide To Managing Stress

Published by

Smart Guide Publications, Inc.
2517 Deer Chase Drive
Norman, OK 73071
www.smartguidepublications.com

For information, address: Smart Guide Publications, Inc. 2517 Deer Creek Drive, Norman, OK 73071

SMART GUIDE and Design are registered trademarks licensed to Smart Guide Publications, Inc.

International Standard Book Number: 978-1-937636-26-5

Library of Congress Catalog Card Number:
11 12 13 14 15   10 9 8 7 6 5 4 3 2 1

Printed in the United States of America

Cover design: Lorna Llewellyn
Copy Editor: Ruth Strother
Back cover design: Joel Friedlander, Eric Gelb, Deon Seifert
Back cover copy: Eric Gelb, Deon Seifert
Illustrations: James Balkovek
Production: Zoë Lonergan
Indexer: Cory Emberson
V.P./Business Manager: Cathy Barker

TESTIMONIALS

"Dr. Robinson provides a detailed roadmap to understanding the nature of mild to severe stresses, the many sources of internal and external stress, and effective processes to deal successfully with them all. This book should be by the bedside of everyone."

—Harville Hendrix, Ph.D., author of *Getting the Love You Want: A Guide for Couples*

"This guide for managing stress gives us powerful tools for navigating anxiety and reactivity. With great clarity and warmth, Bryan Robinson opens us to the possibility of living with an increasing sense of balance, happiness, and ease. This book is an accomplishment! It will be deeply helpful to many."

—Tara Brach, Ph.D., author of *Radical Acceptance: Embracing Your Life with the Heart of a Buddha*

"This simple yet profound guide takes the stress out of managing stress, offering clear information and concrete advice on how to have a calmer, more peaceful life."

—Kristin Neff, Ph.D., author of *Self-Compassion: Stop Beating Yourself Up and Leave Insecurity Behind*

"A rich and thorough guide—the insights on workaholism, addiction, and stress offer especially valuable insights for getting our most critical and insidious risk factors under control."

—Martin Rossman, M.D., author of *The Worry Solution: Using Breakthrough Brain Science to Turn Stress and Anxiety into Confidence and Happiness*

"*The Smart Guide to Managing Stress* is sure to become another best-seller for Bryan Robinson. Readers will love the special features, and Robinson is always the master who can create a step-by-step approach to life-changing actions. Every reader will love Bryan's tips, 'truths' and concepts and find themselves savoring all the wisdom shared in this masterpiece."

—Joy Miller, Ph.D., CEO of Joy Miller & Associates, Counseling and Wellness, author and motivational speaker

"Using easy-to-understand language, this practical book can help virtually anyone to become less stressed. Providing insight into the many causes of stress in modern life, it offers wide-ranging solutions based on the latest research and clinical practices. Dr. Robinson helps us deal more effectively with all aspects of our lives, showing us how to be happier, healthier, and more content, regardless of our circumstances."

—Ronald D. Siegel, Psy.D., Assistant Clinical Professor of Psychology, Harvard Medical School and author of *The Mindfulness Solution: Everyday Practices for Everyday Problems*

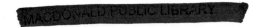

"With humor and authority, Bryan Robinson brings you the latest breakthrough science in clearly written practical tips and exercises."

—Fred Luskin, Ph.D., Director of the Stanford University Forgiveness Project and author of *Forgive for Good*

"*The Smart Guide to Managing Stress* is sure to become the go-to-source for busy individuals seeking a healthier, more productive, and contented life. Dr. Robinson provides an eye-opening and thoughtful 360-degree view on how stress impacts every facet of one's life."

—Chuck Runyon, Co-founder & CEO of Anytime Fitness and coauthor of *Working Out Sucks*

"Bryan Robinson's Guide offers many helpful and creative suggestions for living more sanely—and even thriving—in the midst of the ever-escalating pressures of 21st-century life. He is truly a Doctor of Calm!"

—Sharon Salzberg, Ph.D., author of *Real Happiness: The Power of Meditation, a 28-Day Program* and *Lovingkindness*

"*The Smart Guide to Managing Stress* is an outstanding and exhaustive "must-read" resource for anyone trying to deal more effectively with stress. It provides thorough review of the research and gives excellent and easy-to-follow advice on managing stress."

—Andrew Newberg, M.D., coauthor of *How God Changes Your Brain*

DEDICATION

This book is for my lifelong partner, Jamey McCullers, for your steadfast patience, support, and enduring love.

PERMISSIONS

The Social Readjustment Rating Scale in Chapter 2 was reprinted from *Journal of Psychosomatic Research*, volume 11(issue 2), Thomas Holmes and Richard Rahe. The Social Readjustment Rating Scale, pages 213–218, 1967, with permission from Elsevier.

An Autobiography in Five Short Chapters in Chapter 21, copyright © 1993 from the book *There's a Hole in My Sidewalk* by Portia Nelson. Reprinted with permission of Beyond Words Publishing, Inc., Hillsboro, Oregon. All rights reserved.

ACKNOWLEDGMENTS

I'd like to thank Jamey McCullers for giving me the gift of "seeing the water I'm swimming in" and helping me find the flip side of the stressful life I was stuck in. I'd also like to acknowledge Pema Chodrin and His Holiness the Dalai Lama—both of whom have inspired me by their teachings and being in their presence.

Special gratitude is due to my agent, Sally McMillan, for standing by my side through many ups and downs in the publishing world and for encouraging me to take on this project. I appreciate the technical help of Greg Mayer of Charlotte Street Computers for bailing me out of many computer glitches, Charlie Covington for creating a beautiful website, and Peter at Purplecat for keeping my website alive. And I am eternally indebted to my talented friend, well-known photographer Jon Michael Riley for the time, energy, and creativity he spent on the book photograph.

A hearty "thank you" to my personal trainer, Tricia Thompson, of Anytime Fitness in Asheville, North Carolina, for contributing the information on stretching and Pilates, and to Stephanie Wilder for her editorial assistance on several of the early chapters.

I owe a special debt to my close friends and loved ones who staunchly cover my back and nurture me on an ongoing basis: Sara Thompson; Nancy Chase; Sohnie Luckhardt; Jamey McCullers; Anne Bergeron; Karen DuBose; Rick Werner; Glenda and James Loftin; Blake, Shere, and Nick Loftin; and Stephanie Wilder.

I offer many bows and blessings to the experts who read the unedited manuscript and gave it two thumbs up: Tara Brach; Harville Hendrix; Sharon Salzberg; Andrew Newberg; Kristin Neff; Joy Miller; Ronald Siegel, Martin Rossman, Chuck Runyon, and Fred Luskin.

To all the staff at Smart Guide Publications for their support and cooperation in transforming the manuscript into a book and for their steadfastness in getting the Smart Guide project launched against many roller-coaster obstacles.

Last but not least, I'd like to thank the hundreds, perhaps thousands, of clients and readers of my previous books. As my teachers, you have inspired me with your strength, hope, courage, and resilience on life's sometimes stressful path.

TABLE OF CONTENTS

PART FOUR: *Stress and Your Psychological Health* 169

14 Stress-Buffering Your Mind's Negativity 171

15 Outwitting Stress by Changing Your Thinking 183

INTRODUCTION

In the still lonely hours before dawn, Sara Martin plops in her armchair, grabs a fistful of hair, and stares out the window at the black sky—thoughts racing, heart pounding. Another sleepless night with her mortgage past due, and she just got laid off from her job because of a faltering economy.

Jared Powell zooms down the highway, pounding the steering wheel. The slam of his heartbeat against his chest reminds him that he is late for his presentation. His navigation system had just sent him in the wrong direction on the freeway. After a few dropped calls to notify his boss that he was running late, Jared—sweaty, shaky, frantic—wails at the traffic and shakes his fist at the heavens.

Stress is on the rise for millions of Americans. We live in a rapidly changing, turbulent world in which many of us are trying to hold that line between calm and stressful activity. In the twenty-first century, life is moving faster. With more things to do, the number of hours in the day seem to be shrinking. Plus our technologically driven culture has erased the boundaries that once protected private time, spinning our lives into a blur of constant *doing*, eclipsing our ability to *be*.

Everyone has stress of some sort, and it comes in all shapes and sizes: hassles, worries, pressures, demands, deadlines. They can literally make you sick. Studies have shown that job burnout can cause you to catch the flu, the stress of splitting up with the love of your life makes you more vulnerable to viruses, and long-held anger and resentment have been linked to cancer.

Stress is how you respond when life places demands upon you. You've heard the old expression, "How is life treating you?" On some days it feels like when it rains, it pours. *Stress management* is how you cope with the demands that life lays at your feet (I often ask a client, "How are you treating life?").

Although there's no stress escape hatch, the good news is that not all stress is bad. Without some stress, we wouldn't get a lot done. Think about that extra burst of adrenaline that helps you make a favorable presentation at work or a grand slam to win a baseball game. So stress can actually be positive. In fact, some of the most memorable moments of our lives contain stress: moving into your first house, the day you get married, the birth of your child. On the other hand, when you're constantly running in emergency mode, stress takes a toll on your mind and body. But the other good news is that modern science has given us more effective ways of managing stress than ever before. So once you've accepted that stress is a fact of life and everyone has it, you're on the road to managing it. And that's what this book is all about.

How to Use This Book

You're holding in your hands the most authoritative, up-to-date book on managing stress. This common-sense guide is brimming with chunks of information on the nature of stress, how you can identify it, and what you can do to reduce most of it, manage the rest, and live a healthy, productive, stress-free life. Some stress comes from life circumstances and some from our own self creation. As you read this book, think about your own stress pattern, noticing how much comes from outside and how much from the inside.

I have included a number of special features to guide you on your journey to outsmarting stress. These special features, sprinkled throughout the chapters, provide common-sense methods to help you understand, digest, and apply stress solutions to your everyday life:

➤ *Bulleted Lists:* Essential information is broken down into sound bites that trim the fat and make points clear and easy to follow.

➤ *Quizzes:* Self-tests personalize your journey throughout the book as you assess your unique stressors and find practical solutions.

➤ *Shock Absorbers:* Action-oriented practices and exercises give you a step-by-step approach to stress-proof your life, face difficult challenges, and buffer stressful situations.

➤ *Trending Now From the Smart Files:* Brief facts and statistics (e.g., numbers, percentages) on stress and stress management let you see how you compare with other Americans under stress.

➤ *Recharging Your Batteries:* Bite-sized tips encourage you to pause and reflect on your stress pattern, look at a situation in a different way, and navigate ups and downs with more ease and confidence.

➤ *Truth Serum:* Easy-to-follow highlights from the latest scientific studies on stress and stress management, showing tried and true tools for stress reduction.

➤ *The Doctor of Calm Is In:* Advice and tips from Dr. Bryan employing the stress-reduction theme of "outsmarting your stress" based on my many years of clinical practice and evidence-based research.

➤ *Case Scenarios:* Brief stories of real people (as with Sara Martin and Jared Powell above), depicting a variety of real-life stressors along with practical solutions they take to solve them.

Ready to get rid of some of that stress? Let's get started right now.

PART ONE

The Nature of Stress and Stress Management

CHAPTER 1

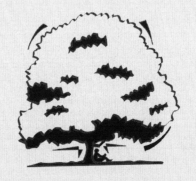

Face-to-Face with Stress as a Fact of Life

In This Chapter

➤ What stress is

➤ Your stress response

➤ Your body under stress

➤ How stress can make you sick

In this chapter, you'll come eyeball-to-eyeball with stress as a fact of life. You'll discover what stress is and how it affects you mentally and physically. You'll gain an understanding of the stress response. And you'll learn how to take your stress temperature, keep a stress journal, and cultivate a different attitude toward your stressors.

Don't Mess Around with Stress

There are some things you just don't mess around with. Like that old Jim Croce song says:

You don't tug on Superman's cape / you don't spit into the wind / you don't pull the mask off that old Lone Ranger / and you don't mess around with Jim.

And there's one more don't to add to the list: You don't mess with stress because it's more powerful than you and me, it's always around, it loves a good fight, and it always wins. Plus, stress can make you miserable, destroy relationships, and it can kill. You can't get rid of it because it's a fact of life and it's here to stay. Fortunately, there's a lot you can do to manage stress.

What Is Stress?

Is your stomach in knots lately? Are you dog tired, dragging yourself through the day? Do you grind your teeth or clench your hands into fists? Are your muscles and joints sore or painful? Do little things set you off more than usual? And did you swear at the car that cut you off on the way to work? If so, you're feeling the effects of stress—the feelings you get when you have to handle more than you're used to or think you're capable of. Stress management is how you cope with the demands that life lays at your feet.

Stress Vocab

Stress is the feeling you get when you're facing demands that exceed your mental, physical, or financial ability to cope and your body has a biochemical response to these perceived threats.

Stress Isn't a Death Sentence

Not long ago, stress might've felt like a death sentence. Not anymore. If you're stressed out, it's not the end of the road. And you're not alone. Everyone has stress of some sort.

Nearly half of Americans say their stress level has risen over the last five years. The truth is that stress is a normal part of life and is with you 24/7. And it comes in all shapes and sizes: hassles, worries, pressures, losses, demands, and deadlines, to name a few.

The encouraging news is that thanks to the advancement of science by our stress forefathers, we have more stress-busting tools at our fingertips than ever before. And there's a lot we can do to reduce most of it, manage the rest, and live a long, healthy, productive, stress-free life.

Truth Serum

The concept of stress and many of the stress reduction techniques that I discuss in this book wouldn't exist if it weren't for Hans Selye, known as the father of stress. He was an Austrian endocrinologist who in 1936 first coined the term *stress* and identified the stress response. His research demonstrates how the body manufactures its own poisons when under siege by stressful events—whether positive (good stress such as buying a new house) or negative (bad stress such as too much debt).

Let's start with some statistics. Knowing stress statistics and facts can help you understand how your stress compares to others. The way experts know how stress affects you and me is through surveys, opinion polls, face-to-face interviews, and controlled research studies. The sidebar showcases a few of these findings. How many apply to you?

Trending Now from the Smart Files

➤ A National Health Interview Survey shows that 75 percent of the American public experience some stress at least once every two weeks.

➤ A 2007 American Psychological Association poll reveals that although 82 percent of Americans handle stress well, half say they're having problems with their physical and mental health and work and relationship pressures.

➤ The Higher Education Research Institute reports that overwhelming stress and financial pressures caused the percentage of emotionally healthy college students to drop from 64 percent in 1985 to 52 percent in 2010.

Common Stressors that Can Flip You Out

Sometimes it can feel like stress is coming at you from all angles, especially with the lightning speed of the world we live in. Pressures come from work woes, relationship problems, money worries, parenting concerns, overcrowding, and waiting. Plus, with all the technology we depend on, the breakdown of your machines can send you over the edge. Here are just a few examples of stressors that can make you sizzle:

> ➤ Your computer crashes

> ➤ Someone cuts you off in traffic

> ➤ Bills are piling up

> ➤ Long, slow-moving lines

> ➤ It's 100 degrees and your air conditioner is on the blink

> ➤ The kids are driving you up the wall

> ➤ Your partner or spouse makes plans without consulting you

> ➤ You're overloaded at work

➤ Your boss chews you out

➤ You've waited in the doctor's office for over an hour

➤ Your neighbor's Lady Gaga CD rumbles into the wee hours

➤ You dropped your cell phone into the toilet

Your Stress Response: A Doozy of a Safety Scanner

When besieged by stress, your body is prewired to kick into red alert to keep you safe. This is called the stress response. Your brain constantly scans your inner and outer worlds for threats. Once it registers situations as threatening, your stress response automatically fires up. Your autonomic nervous system (ANS) sends emergency instructions to the rest of your body. These messages cause your body to amp up salivation, sweating, heart rate, breathing, and digestion to help you survive danger.

Stress Vocab

Autonomic nervous system (ANS) is the part of your nervous system that regulates your internal organs not under your conscious control such as heart rate, respiration, blood flow, digestion, even sweat and saliva.

The Neurochemical Cocktail that Marinates You

When you're frazzled, your brain acts as an internal slingshot, pumping a cocktail of stress hormones into your bloodstream. Your body stews in its cortisol and adrenaline juices. Your chest heaves, heart rate jumps, blood pressure leaps, respiration rate skyrockets, and muscles tighten, readying you for action.

Stress Vocab

Cortisol is a stress hormone secreted by the adrenal glands that regulates blood pressure and energy for your body.

Glucose (sugar) levels spike to give you energy. Your body's quick reactions make your blood flow faster so that it can deliver more oxygen to your muscles. This gives your body the strength it needs to fight or flee from a threatening situation. Your brain tells your body to stay in this alert state until it's convinced the threat is over. Once the threat passes, your body returns to its normal functioning.

Truth Serum

A Yale University study found that under threat even insects like grasshoppers—that normally feed on protein such as grasses—switch to munching on sugary goldenrod plants. The sugary foods provide fuel to quickly feed their amped-up bodies in case they need to flee. When you're stressed out, your cortisol production kicks in. Then your metabolism speeds up, and you, too, are more likely to seek out digested sugars, fats, and carbs for a quick energy boost. No wonder we're a nation of stressed-out fast-food addicts!

So That's Why I Crave Pizza!

Middle-aged creep isn't the jerk in a trench coat leaning over your shoulder with his camera phone—it's the added spare tire, usually caused by stress, that refuses to budge no matter how much you diet or exercise. When you're upset, the fats and sugars you eat go straight to your belly. These fat deposits make you even more vulnerable to stress, and your body secretes even more glucose. That jacks up your craving for sweets and fat. And boom! Fat is stored in your belly again, throwing you into a chicken-and-egg cycle.

Under stress, you'll find it difficult, but not impossible, to maintain healthy balance: healthy eating habits, ample sleep, and exercise are usually the first to go down the toilet. The more stressed you are, the more you eat, the more weight you gain, and the more you skimp on exercise. Increased weight makes you more stressed and exhausted. Weight gain and lethargy are stress symptoms that weaken your ability to cope, making you more susceptible to daily pressures.

Fight-or-Flight Mode

You could be stressed for reasons from your genetic past. At one time, your primitive fight-or-flight response would have switched on at breakneck speed to help you survive attacks from other tribes and wild animals. But you don't have to worry about attacks from lions or tigers anymore (unless you work in a zoo). Still, your brain and body carry the reflex of these old fears before you step up to the podium, altar, or counseling session with your spouse—a flip-flop in the stomach, a skipping heartbeat, a tightness in your shoulders.

Everyday Threats

Nowadays your fight-or-flight response revs up your heartbeat, jump-starts your breathing, tightens your muscles, and pumps a burst of energy to help you fend off danger or "get the heck out of Dodge" in the middle of a bank robbery, car wreck, or house fire.

Stress Vocab

Fight-or-Flight Response is your nervous system's automatic chemical reaction to threats so that you can fight off or run away from threatening situations.

But your nervous system can't tell the difference between life-and-death situations and psychological dangers. So your body responds the same way to any stressful event to minimize your losses and maximize your gains. You might notice a rise in stress juices if your job is threatened, your calendar is jammed, your partner or spouse is upset with you, or you're having trouble paying your mortgage. "What if I can't find a job?" "What if she breaks up with me?" "What if I can't pay my bills?" To your brain, these situations feel just as dangerous as a wild bear attack.

Shock Absorber

Do the jitters pole-vault into your life before a big job interview, medical diagnosis, or confrontation with a loved one? Uninvited stress jolts your fight-or-flight mode because your brain is constantly on the lookout for threats. Your body reacts with an automatic stress response so that you can overcome big hurdles. Cortisol and adrenaline squirts propel you into action, making you fidget like you've had a six-pack of Red Bull. You sweat; your mouth goes dry. Your body's energy is diverted to your limbs to put you in action mode. And blood flow is redirected from your digestive tract to your muscles, leaving you with butterflies or nausea.

As your muscles tense in preparedness, you might notice tightness, even cramps or spasms. Healthy nutrition, brisk exercise, and a good night's sleep will offset the jitters. And deep, slow breathing can cushion the jitters before your big moment. But a properly framed attitude is the best shock absorber. So in the heat of the moment, remember: your jitters are not working against you; they are working for you in your mind and body's natural way of protecting you from harm.

Imagined Threats

Perceived threats can cause your nervous system to respond as if you're in danger even if you're not. Suppose the security alarm in your house goes off. You don't know if there's a real intruder or if somebody accidentally tripped the alarm. But your body responds the same regardless. Your stress response jolts into emergency mode. It pumps stress hormones into your bloodstream to protect you from real or imagined threats and throws you into full-out battle or hasty retreat.

Subtle threats also can trigger your stress response. A frown from your boss across the conference table; a frustrated tone from your spouse or partner; rolling eyes and lifted brow from a coworker; a cold shrug when you try to hug your teenager. You can feel the stress hormones pulsating through your veins.

After the danger is over, your body returns to its natural resting state. But for people living under prolonged stress, such as caring for an ailing adult parent, the stress alarm doesn't shut off. The longer it stays on, the harder it is to shut off, and the greater the toll on your mind and body.

Truth Serum

Can you catch a cold just because you split with the love of your dreams? Can job stress cause you to get the flu? Can long-held resentments give you cancer? Think of how many times you've felt worried, stressed out, or depressed only to have those feelings followed by a cold or other virus. The World Health Organization lists stress as the number one health problem in the world. And it's no wonder. On the outside you might rant and rave, freeze in fear, or get away when you're stressed out. But there's a lot going on inside your body that you might not be aware of. And the longer you stay in fight-or-flight mode, the harder it is to get out of it and the more damage it does to your body. Prolonged stress can trigger everything from headaches, eczema, and psoriasis to heart attack and cancer.

Your Stress Boomerang Will Come Back and Could Make You Sick (Ah Choo!)

Scientists say that almost any thought that enters your mind finds its way into the body. Your cells eavesdrop on your thoughts 24/7. And you become the recipient of the biochemical effects of your own worry, frustration, or rage. When you harbor anger or resentment, you literally turn them inward upon yourself, where they can harm you emotionally and physically.

A negative reaction to someone who doesn't meet your standards of perfection, for example, boomerangs back to you on the inside. Do you have a chronic habit of getting upset when things don't go your way? If so, your emotions can set off a chemical chain reaction. Like a boomerang, your body unleashes stress enzymes that can compromise your immune system, damage your heart, and cause gastrointestinal disorders—all in an effort to respond to perceived threats. Prolonged threats are even linked to biochemical changes in your body that can produce cancerous cells.

Stress Vocab

T-cells are white blood cells that play a major role in immunity by protecting your body from disease and infections.

Shock Absorber

Positive thoughts and feelings create body chemistry that boosts your health. Laughter and optimism are shock absorbers; they strengthen your immune system by increasing the number of disease-fighting immune cells. They inoculate you with interleukins and interferons, powerful cancer-fighting enzymes. Plus, humor and lightheartedness activate endorphins that reduce stress, ease pain, and brighten your outlook. When you embrace lightheartedness and look for the silver lining, you put the brakes on the negative effects of stress, stay healthier, and live longer. So catch a funny movie, check out a comedy club, or share a laugh.

Stress and Your Immune System

The constant bombardment of stress hormones from moodiness, anxiety, or depression disrupts your body's biochemical balance. It weakens your immune system, giving a free pass to infection, illness, and disease. You become more susceptible to colds, flu, and other viruses. Studies show that couples undergoing separation or divorce have a lower T-cell count than couples in strong marriages because of accompanying stress. Prolonged stress can also lead to type 2 diabetes, cancer, and autoimmune diseases such as rheumatoid arthritis.

Stress and Your Heart

After a while, chronic stress can lead to high blood pressure, heart disease, and even heart attack. Too much adrenaline blocks the cell's ability to clear dangerous cholesterol from your bloodstream. An elevated cholesterol level makes platelets stickier, clogging arteries, damaging their inner lining, and precipitating heart attacks. Chronic stress creates plaque buildup twice as fast in your arteries, causing them to constrict, reducing blood flow to the heart.

Stress and Gastrointestinal Problems

Stress wreaks havoc on your digestive system. It slows down your digestion because your brain notifies your body to redirect blood flow to your muscles to cope with the stressful situation. The digestive disruption can leave your stomach in knots or cause constipation, gas, and bloating. And it aggravates other digestive disorders such as irritable bowel syndrome and colitis. Studies also show that under stressful conditions you are more likely to have gastroesopheal reflux disease (GERD)—increased stomach acid that travels back up to your esophagus.

Stress Vocab

Endorphins are brain chemicals known as neurotransmitters that act like your body's natural pain killers and stress fighters and induce peaceful feelings.

The Pace You Keep

When you add adrenaline-fueled rushing and hurrying to the mix, you have double trouble. Grabbing fast food and chugging Red Bulls and Starbucks on the run further contribute to your bad physical and mental health. Look at the number of TV commercials for acid relief, headaches, muscle soreness, hypertension, and mood relaxers. Studies show that the stress hormones your body produces from constant hurrying and rushing act like speed, revving you up and making you restless and easily agitated, unable to relax during downtime.

Sideswiped by stress, you tense your muscles to brace against it. And you get angry at yourself for not seeing it coming. Or you ignore it altogether. After a period of neglecting your body's stress signals, you become overly reactive to normal stressors. And you have difficulty handling minor situations that used to be a piece of cake. The end result is a short-circuiting of your body functions, daily routines, job performance, and relationships. This is the equivalent of not checking the gauges on your dashboard and ending up with a major engine malfunction.

Your Body Has a Mind of Its Own

It's as if your body has a mind of its own, tensing and tightening in reaction to the daily grind. The human body is wired to "think" for you so that you can survive while managing the big picture of your life—like paying bills, managing your portfolio, picking up the kids from school, or burning the midnight oil to meet a deadline.

Your body is constantly responding to life's stressors while you're busy with other pursuits. For example, when I have a deadline, I often notice my shoulders hunched up to my ears in reaction to the pressure. Now that I've become more aware of my shoulders' tendency to contract, I make a concerted effort to keep those muscles relaxed.

When you don't listen and take care of your body, it will grab your attention by speaking to you in a stern voice: headaches, indigestion, muscle spasms, body aches and pains, clenched jaw, a glitch in your hitch. But when you become better acquainted with your body, listen to it and take care of it, you'll notice a huge drop in your stress level.

Truth Serum

Physician Jon Kabat-Zinn developed a mindfulness-based stress reduction (MBSR) program in 1979 at the University of Massachusetts Medical Center. His eight-week program helps patients, failed by conventional medicine, reduce their stress-related illnesses. Through evidence-based research, he has shown that mindfulness enhances well-being and treats stress-related conditions ranging from chronic pain to breast and prostate cancer. I'll discuss mindfulness in detail and show you how to apply some of these techniques in Chapter 12.

The "Write" Way to Face Your Stress

A good way to become familiar with your stress pattern is to start a stress journal. Did you know that jotting down your thoughts, feelings, worries, frustrations, and stressors can actually improve your health? Studies show that writing out stressful experiences has positive physiological payoffs: enhanced immune system, reduction in severity of illness, and mental release of past disturbing events.

Advantages of a Stress Journal

You can reap many benefits from keeping a journal of your stressful experiences:

➤ Availability: Your stress journal can be your silent friend, available anytime of the day and in the wee hours of the morning when friends, health care providers, or support systems might not be around.

➤ Release: A stress journal is an outlet for you to let go of your feelings. You can vent your worry, anger, hurt, frustration, or sadness without fear of judgment, reprisal, or censure. And you don't have to apologize or worry about hurting someone's feelings.

➤ Insight: Your stress journal gives you insight into your stress triggers and your reactions to them. It keeps track of repeated stressors in the course of your day. And it pinpoints how you handle pressure and areas where you can develop better coping skills.

➤ Progress: Your stress journal provides a permanent map of the progress you make in dealing with stress over time.

Your Stress Needle

One way to map your stress is with what I call your stress needle. When I treat clients for stress, I start by asking them to tell me how stressed they feel. I use the 10-point scale below where 0 is no stress, or neutral, and 10 is the highest stress you can imagine. This scale is a great way to get a clearer picture of where your stress is and measure how it changes over time. You can record those changes in your stress journal for a permanent progress report.

0 1 2 3   4 5 6 7   8 9 10

(no stress/neutral)   (moderate stress)   (highest stress)

Recharging Your Batteries

You can take your stress temperature by asking how stressful you feel right now on a scale from 0 to 10. You can also recall times when you were under stress and compare those to how you feel now. Plus, you can use this measurement to identify stress patterns by comparing your ratings as they go up or down from one situation to another. The comparison gives you an indication of what types of events trigger your stress. Your stress needle might be at a 3 right now, but it might've been a 7 or 8 last week when you made that presentation at work. In situations where your needle is high, think about some simple strategies that will lower it. Deep breathing is one that I'll show you in later chapters, along with loads of other stress prevention and management techniques.

Getting Started

Your stress journal belongs to you and you alone. So make it convenient for your personal use. And keep your entries brief; one or two sentences will do. If you're using a computer, make sure you password protect your entries so you can be honest with your feelings.

In future chapters, I'll suggest exercises for you to note in your journal. It's up to you to decide if these suggestions are relevant for your particular situation and whether or not you want to take the time to record them.

Even more important is for you to keep an ongoing personal record of times you feel pressured. You can take your stress temperature and record how you feel in the morning compared to later in the day. This will tell you if your mood sours as the day drags on and if so, what event triggers the shift. Plus, noting specific situations or people you avoid during the day can help you figure out what threatens you. You'll start to identify patterns and themes that give you insight into your comfortable stress temperature and what unpleasant situations you need to change.

Tips on What to Record

Here are some points to record in your stress journal:

➤ What was the stressor? (I was behind on my deadline)

➤ What feelings did you have? (worry, frustration)

➤ What were your thoughts? (I'm gonna get fired)

➤ How did your body respond? (sick to my stomach)

➤ What action did you take? (I threw an all-nighter to finish)

➤ What action would you take next time? (I'll get started earlier instead of procrastinating)

As you can see from my example, a stress journal can help you understand the sources of your stress and how you can handle them. Plus, the insight you gain can point you to coping skills that will prevent or reduce your stress in the future.

Accept Stress in My Life? Seriously?

In this book, I won't tell you to put up your dukes to beat stress or use words like *combat*, *battle*, *conquer*, or *fight* as a strategy to manage stress. An adversarial relationship between you and your stressors can lead to greater frustration and anxiety. But an accepting attitude can help you lower your stress needle. "What? Are you on crack?" I can hear you gasp. I realize it sounds counterintuitive, but hold on. Don't "de-friend" me just yet. Consider the idea that war is stressful and fighting stress can do more harm than good—even raise your stress needle. This book is not about going to war with stress; it's about outsmarting it. Once you accept stress as a fact of life, you're already on the road to de-stressing, relaxing, and managing daily pressures.

The Doctor Of Calm Is In

Nothing has changed but my attitude; everything has changed

—Anthony de Mello

My prescription: Check your attitude toward stress and the language you use to manage it once or twice daily or until your stress temperature drops and your combative frame of mind subsides. If symptoms persist, continue reading on for further remedy. On second thought, read on regardless and learn how to send stress packing. Here's to outsmarting your stress!

CHAPTER 2

When Stress Hits Home

In This Chapter

> The signposts of stress

> Your stress profile

> Sources of stress

> Types of stress

In this chapter, you'll discover what stressors afflict most Americans and what your own signs of stress are. You'll distinguish between external stressors and those that result from the perspective you take. You'll identify the different types of stress and how your body responds to good and bad types. As you understand the sources of your own stress, you'll see that you have more control over it than you think.

Recognizing the Signposts of Stress

Now that you have an understanding of what stress is and how it affects your body, you might be wondering what

Truth Serum

The American Psychological Association wanted to know what stresses people out. In a 2007 survey, one of the most thorough polls to date, the organization asked thousands of ordinary Americans about their stress symptoms. Then they classified the answers into two types: physical symptoms such as digestive problems and psychological symptoms such as mood swings. They found that:

> 77 percent of the population has physical symptoms

> 73 percent have psychological symptoms

stress looks like and how it shows up in your everyday life. It's probably safe to say that you've had your share of stress and already know some of the signs. But if you're like many busy people today, you've learned to ignore and push through them. Paying attention to these signals is the first step in reducing your stress.

What Are Your Stress Signals?

How do you know if you're stressed? It's possible for you to be stressed and not realize it. Knowing the signs raises your awareness and helps you manage it. Stress symptoms show up in people in different ways. You might have physical, mental, emotional, or social signs. To get a better picture of your stress symptoms, check out the list below for some common signs. Put a check mark beside each symptom you've noticed in the past month.

Physical Stress:

- ➤ Accident prone
- ➤ Fatigue
- ➤ Headache
- ➤ Insomnia
- ➤ Muscle tension and soreness
- ➤ Pounding heart
- ➤ Restlessness
- ➤ Shortness of breath
- ➤ Skin rashes such as eczema
- ➤ Teeth grinding
- ➤ Upset stomach
- ➤ Weight change

_____Total Physical Stress Score

Mental Stress:

- ➤ Boredom
- ➤ Confusion at home
- ➤ Confusion at work
- ➤ Decline in problem solving
- ➤ Dulling of the senses
- ➤ Errors in judgment

➤ Forgetfulness

➤ Loss of creativity

➤ Lowered productivity

➤ Mental exhaustion

➤ Negative attitude

➤ Poor concentration skills

_____Total Mental Stress Score

Emotional Stress:

➤ Anxiety

➤ Bad temper

➤ Constant worrying

➤ Crying spells

➤ Depression

➤ Easily discouraged

➤ Feeling uptight

➤ Irritability

➤ Loss of sense of humor

➤ Mood swings

➤ Nervous laughter

➤ Self-criticism

_____Total Emotional Stress Score

Social Stress:

➤ Being impatient

➤ Being vindictive

➤ Clamming up

➤ Isolation

➤ Lashing out at coworkers

➤ Lashing out at family

➤ Lashing out at friends

➤ Loneliness

➤ Lowered sex drive

➤ Lying

➤ Nagging others

➤ Resentment of others

_____Total Social Stress Score

A Profile of Your Stress Symptoms

Your stress profile can help you pinpoint the area of your life in which stress symptoms show up most. Do you have physical, mental, emotional, or social stress? Or do you have a combination of all four?

➤ Tally check marks in each of the four areas and write the sum in the Total Score blank.

➤ Transfer each score onto the appropriate blank on the stress grid. Put an *X* on the line above each stress symptom that matches your score. For example, if your physical stress score is six, put an *X* on the vertical line that is across from the number six.

➤ Repeat this step for your mental, emotional, and social stress scores.

Your Stress Grid

12

11

10

9

8

7

6

5

4

3

2

1

0 _____

       Physical   Mental   Emotional   Social

Scores   _____   _____   _____   _____

Shock Absorber

As you review your scores on the stress grid, what symptoms are most common? And in which of the four areas do you need to focus attention first to reduce the symptoms? In your stress journal, record small ways you can prevent or reduce symptoms in the four areas. For example, if you have a high score in physical symptoms, a massage might help you relax. Or if you scored high in emotional symptoms, you might consider some of the relaxation techniques that I discuss in later chapters. As you read on, you'll discover tons of tips to help you manage your stress symptoms. But for now, consult your primary health care professional for any symptoms that you're concerned about. Your medical provider is the best person to advise you on what your symptoms mean and what action you should take.

What Sends You Off the Launch Pad?

Now, let's get to exactly what makes you feel like screaming, "I've had it up to here!" You might already know. Your answer might be different from mine or the average person's because what you consider stressful might not be perceived as stressful by someone else. A 2007 national survey by the American Psychological Association (APA) found out what typical Americans said their biggest stressors are. Check out what they discovered and see how your personal stressors compare with their findings:

➤ Financial pressures

➤ Health problems

➤ Work strain

Financial Pressures

In the survey, 73 percent listed finances as the number one factor affecting their stress level, rising to 75 percent in a 2011 APA follow-up study. The typical American has problems making ends meet with rising costs and slimmer paychecks. If you've ever been under financial pressure, you know the worry and anxiety and perhaps even the desperation that can lead to working multiple jobs or longer hours—actions that add another layer of stress.

Health Problems

A total of 70 percent of women and 63 percent of men say they are stressed over health problems affecting their families. They cite physical problems such as upset stomach, change in appetite, muscle tension, and fatigue. And they list emotional problems such as irritability, anger, nervousness, and lack of energy.

Trending Now from the Smart Files

Here are some sources of work stress:

➤ 61 percent of workers report heavy workloads

➤ 57 percent of women and 55 percent of men cite worries about job stability

➤ 54 percent of workers say health problems cause stress

➤ 45 percent of workers list job insecurity

➤ 25 percent of workers have taken a mental health day to cope with stress

Source: American Psychological Association, 2007

Work Strain

In the 2007 survey, 62 percent say their jobs caused them stress, rising to 70 percent in the 2011 APA follow-up study. In a difficult economy, you might find it harder than ever to cope with challenges at work. Job stress is high on the list for most people. The pressures you take with you to work and the ones waiting for you when you get there can lead to overload and burnout: Finding employment in a competitive market, holding on to your position, dealing with your job's unique stressors, worrying about layoffs or budget cuts, working double or triple duty carrying the load of other workers because of job cuts, and coping with climbing the ladder of success—all create stress in the workplace. If you're like most people, you spend a huge chunk of your life working. And if you toil in a high-pressured work environment (whether self-imposed or imposed by your job), it can be a constant drain on your overall life satisfaction.

Other Sources of Stress

Stress comes from a variety of sources that can be divided roughly into two categories: personal stressors and environmental stressors. Environmental stressors include all the challenges, expectations, and hardships you face on a daily basis. Personal stressors include your perceptions of external threats, your unique personality traits that affect how you react, and the coping skills you develop to offset them.

Environmental Stressors

Much of your stress comes from external factors in your life. You have little or no control over some of these factors and some control over others. The list is endless, but here are a few examples of typical environmental stressors:

➤ Unemployment and futility in finding a job

➤ An overly demanding job where budget cuts threaten your position

➤ The aftermath of a tornado or other natural disaster

➤ Mounting bills with no relief in sight

➤ Serious health problems that limit your activities

➤ The dizzying pace of the world around you as you fall behind

➤ Your kids are a handful

➤ A blind date

➤ A golf game

➤ Speaking in public

➤ You're going through a breakup

➤ Inability to keep up with all of your responsibilities

➤ Your house is vandalized

➤ Your neighborhood has a lot of traffic noise

Shock Absorber

Start keeping a record of situations where you feel stress the most: at work, in a relationship, at school, in social situations, in your family. Then pinpoint exactly who or what is stressful about that situation. How do you react? And what are the consequences of your actions?

Using the stress temperature needle from Chapter 1, rate each situation on a scale from 0 to 10. If you rate financial pressure as an 8, make a specific statement about finances that gives a clear picture of why it's stressful for you: "I'm not making enough money to pay my bills." Jot down some actions you can take to relieve stress in each situation—things that don't add more problems to an already stressful situation. Suppose a coworker isn't carrying his weight, and the work falls on you. Perhaps speaking up can make a difference. Or could it be the way you're looking at the problem?

As you read through the book, take your stress temperature from time to time on the stressors you identified, and use your stress journal to map progress as you manage them.

Personal Stressors

Sometimes stress comes from personality traits that heighten your susceptibility to pressure. And sometimes it comes from your perspective—the unique way you perceive and react under pressure. Again, the list is endless, but here are a few examples of self-created stress:

➤ You procrastinate on deadlines and work furiously at the last minute.

➤ You bite off more than you can chew.

➤ You tend to see the glass as half empty instead of half full.

➤ You don't draw a line and say no when you're overloaded.

➤ Little things set you off.

➤ You're easily overwhelmed and tend to worry too much.

➤ You have to be in control of most situations.

➤ You get upset when people don't meet your standards of perfection.

➤ It's difficult for you to ask for help.

➤ You seek approval through pleasing people, which makes it hard to say no.

➤ You're too hard on yourself.

➤ You get upset when things don't go your way.

➤ It's hard to relax and let go.

Shock Absorber

List your three top stressors. Then name one action you can take to manage each of them. Here are a few tips to get you going:

➤ Face the stressor head-on: Tired of a friend's habitual lateness? Speak up.

➤ Take another course of action: Tax deadline stressing you out? Prepare earlier.

➤ Avoid the stressor: Scared of heights? Avoid high places.

➤ Change your outlook: Upset over a fender bender? Be glad no one was hurt and you have insurance to pay for repairs.

Types of Stress

Now that you're somewhat familiar with your stress symptoms and the many sources of stress, I'd like to introduce you to the various types of stress. You might not know it but stress has many faces, and it even has a good side. But the more debilitating types of stress make you want to sign up for the witness protection program and disappear into an anonymous life far away. Let's start with the good stress.

Good Stress

How many times have you had that sinking feeling before giving a presentation to coworkers or facing someone over a relationship spat? Sometimes stress feels like one of those cruel ghosts that haunts you day and night, stalking you on a pressure-cooker day, lurking over your shoulder while you're pitching ideas to clients or stretching your dollars to make ends meet. If you're like most people, you might think of stress as an enemy infiltrator. You ignore it, get frustrated with it, or try to extinguish it.

In some ways, stress has gotten a bum rap, but it's not all bad. In fact, good stress is so common that Hans Selye gave it the name eustress in the 1930s. Eustress is the kind of stress that gets you motivated and lets you know you're fully involved in your life. It helped Tiger Woods win golf games, Lance Armstrong champion his cycling races, and Meryl Streep snag her string of Oscars.

Stress Vocab

Eustress is the term for good stress that motivates you, makes you feel alive, and helps you thrive as you meet life's challenges.

Shock Absorber

A little stress is a good thing, sometimes even a great thing to have. Your brain is actually wired for stress to protect and keep you safe. Like the kick-butt drill sergeant who doesn't want you to get your head blown off in combat, stress warns you of threats, and motivates you to stay on course to do the right thing. It keeps you from making a fool of yourself in front of your peers, exposing yourself to ridicule or embarrassment. If stress didn't keep you on your toes, you might not be as successful in your job; your relationships could crumble, you'd be more susceptible to danger, and your life could fall apart. Plus, you wouldn't have as much fun. Stress gives you that thrill and excitement when you're on a roller coaster, bungee jumping, going on safari, rooting for your Super Bowl team, going to your first prom, getting married, enjoying sex, buying your first house, delivering your first child, going through the haunted house at Halloween. So, developing an attitude of gratitude toward good stress can be a good thing.

Minor Stress

In and of itself minor stress—such as misplacing your cell phone or getting a parking ticket—is simply an annoyance that doesn't take much of a toll on you. But even minor stressors can send you over the edge when they ambush you in rapid-fire succession. It feels like you can't catch a break. After a while, you start to feel as if you're being assaulted and your distress skyrockets.

Case in point: You wake up still tired from a bad night's sleep but manage to drag yourself out of bed. You don't have time for breakfast, and you can't find your car keys. You finally get it together and head for work in the drenching rain. And boom! You have a flat tire that makes you late for an important meeting. After a stampeding string of minor stressors you bang the steering wheel, sneer at motorists spraying you with water, and shake your fist at the Heavens. We've all had days like that. The key is to nip the escalating minor stressors in the bud at the outset before you plummet into a pit of despair.

Quiz

As you read about the different types of stress, think about the types that you struggle with daily. Would you say your stress is mostly minor, acute, or chronic? Or is your life a combination of all three? And how much of your stress would you classify as eustress? Assign percentages to the types of stress you encounter on a daily basis. They will total 100 percent.

- ➤ _____Minor stress
- ➤ _____Acute stress
- ➤ _____Chronic stress
- ➤ _____Eustress
- ➤ <u>100%</u> Total

What do you notice? Does good stress outweigh the bad? Do you have chronic stress? Or is most of it minor? How can you use your observations to pinpoint where to put stress cushions in your life? Record your findings in your stress journal.

Acute Stress

Major life stressors are the earth-shattering changes that rock your world and jolt you into the realization that your life isn't permanent. These are the big kahunas for which you always seem to rise to the occasion, surmounting and adjusting to with time—like job loss, divorce, diagnosis of a terminal illness, or death of a loved one. If you're like most people, you somehow find the strength and courage to face and endure the major life events.

Chronic Stress

Chronic stress is the most dangerous of all stress types because there's no immediate relief. Prolonged stress raises your risk of physical illness: living under constant threat of financial uncertainty, long-term care of a disabled family member, rearing a drug-addicted teenager who is in and out of rehab, trapped in a job you despise, years of unemployment, constant worry about your own or a loved one's health, fear of foreclosure on your house.

A 2012 APA survey found that caregivers of disabled relatives are more likely than the general public to report a higher stress level, increased stress in the past five years, and the development of a chronic illness. Chronic stress doesn't give your body a chance to return to its natural resting state. Imagine what would happen if you left your car engine running for a long time. After a while it would overheat and run out of gas, coughing and sputtering before it shuts down. That's what long-term stress does to your body. Constant stress on your cells produces the hormones adrenaline and cortisol. Over time and in large doses, prolonged stress can be hazardous to your health.

Stress Can Be Hazardous to Your Health

Another way to evaluate the role stress plays in your life is to evaluate its cumulative effects. Regardless of whether your stress is minor, acute, good, or bad, when stressors accumulate, they take a toll on your health. And as you'll see, it's not just what happens to you. The perspective you take also makes a big difference in how you're affected by stress.

Recharging Your Batteries

Scientists say getting outdoors is the ticket to reducing stress and revitalizing your health. Studies show that spending twenty minutes a day outdoors can make you feel peppier. Taking a brisk ten-minute walk raises and sustains your energy level and recalibrates a fatigued brain. Research shows you perform better after a walk in the woods than after a walk along a busy street. So find a park or natural setting. Feel the breeze on your face, notice the colors and smells of leaves and flowers, pay attention to the sounds of chirping crickets, warbling birds, or rushing water.

If you can't get outside, don't fret. Studies show that simply viewing nature can be restorative. So find a window and watch a squirrel scamper up a tree, birds nesting, or a sunset. Connecting with nature transports you out of the artificial world of social media and machines and calms and relaxes you.

Effects of Cumulative Stress

Thomas Holmes and Richard Rahe examined the medical records of over 5,000 patients and found strong links between life events and stress-related illnesses. Their findings consist of forty-three life events that contribute to illness. To find out if events in your life have put you at risk, circle the stress score beside each life event that has occurred in the past year. Then add up each score you circle to get your total stress score. If you're in a committed relationship with a same-sex or opposite-sex partner, treat your relationship as marriage and your partner as spouse in response to the life events. Here's an example: If you were married (50), got pregnant (40), took out a big home mortgage (32), and got slapped with a traffic ticket (11), your total stress score would be 133, which means you only have a slight risk of illness.

- ➤ Death of spouse 100
- ➤ Divorce 73
- ➤ Marital separation 65
- ➤ Jail time 63
- ➤ Death of close family member 63
- ➤ Personal injury or illness 53
- ➤ Marriage 50
- ➤ Fired at work 47
- ➤ Marital reconciliation 45
- ➤ Retirement 45
- ➤ Change in health of family member 44
- ➤ Pregnancy 40
- ➤ Sexual difficulties 39
- ➤ Gain of new family member 39
- ➤ Business readjustment 39
- ➤ Change in financial state 38
- ➤ Death of close friend 37
- ➤ Change to different line of work 36
- ➤ Change in number of arguments with spouse 35
- ➤ A large mortgage or loan 31
- ➤ Foreclosure of mortgage or loan 30
- ➤ Change in responsibilities at work 29

➤ Son or daughter leaving home 29

➤ Trouble with in-laws 29

➤ Outstanding personal achievement 28

➤ Spouse begins or stops work 26

➤ Begin or end school/college 26

➤ Change in living conditions 25

➤ Revision of personal habits 24

➤ Trouble with boss 23

➤ Change in work hours or conditions 20

➤ Change in residence 20

➤ Change in school/college 20

➤ Change in recreation 19

➤ Change in church 19

➤ Change in social activities 18

➤ Moderate loan or mortgage 17

➤ Change in sleeping habits 16

➤ Change in number of family get-togethers 15

➤ Change in eating habits 15

➤ Vacation 13

➤ Christmas 12

➤ Minor violations of the law 11

Your Cumulative Stress Score

Your stress score is a rough measure of how good and bad cumulative stress affects your health. Whatever your score, it's important to remember that your perception of the stressful event and how you coped with it—not just the event itself—determines your risk of illness.

Recharging Your Batteries

As I mentioned in Chapter 1, the more you're able to accept stressful situations, the less stress you'll have. Though the emotional acceptance of stress is not easy, it can create a calm, clear mind for handling pressures. And this ability varies from person to person because people react differently to stressors.

Suppose you're cut off in traffic and you quickly accept it, grateful that your car wasn't banged up and nobody got hurt. But your commute buddy slams his fist on the dashboard and yells an obscenity. Your friend will suffer greater negative consequences than you will.

But suppose the situation is reversed: You're the one who becomes angry and lashes out. When you find yourself forcing, resisting, or clinging to people or situations over which you have no control, take a breath and step back from the stressor. See if you can relax, let go, and accept any aspects of it that you can't change. Then take a calmer course of action that brings more clarity and serenity into your life.

➤ Scores of 300 plus: Your cumulative stress puts you at high or very high risk of illness in the near future.

➤ Scores of 150–299: Your cumulative stress puts you at moderate to high risk of illness in the near future.

➤ Scores of 150 and below: Your cumulative stress puts you in the low to moderate chance of becoming ill in the near future.

So I'm Stressed (Duh!), Now What?

If you find yourself in the high-risk category, keep your life as steady as you can. Try to avoid added stress by avoiding unnecessary changes. You might not be able to control all future stressors, but you can postpone moving, buying a new car, starting a new business, getting married, or taking on new responsibilities. When possible, wait until your life is stable before taking the next stressful plunge so you don't bite off more than you can chew and get "cortisol drenched."

Bourgeois Stress: Is It Worth a Stressfest?

Do you throw a fit when the big game is rained out? Do you scream and beat the steering wheel over airline delays? When you get upset over the small stuff that usually doesn't matter in the scheme of things, you could be having bourgeois stress. Chances are you get so used to living with stress that you have a stressfest over little things. And you might not even realize it. Sometimes asking yourself if a situation is worth stressing over gives you a change of perspective, helps you separate small things from big things, and relieves some of the stress you feel.

"Rx from Dr. Bryan"

The Doctor Of Calm Is In

Men are disturbed not by things, but by the views which they take of them

—Epictetus

My prescription: Ask yourself how important the stressor really is. Better yet, ask yourself if what you're stressing over is truly a stressor or if you are just in the habit of stressing? Continue this remedy daily or until you feel like throwing a party instead of a fit. Here's to outsmarting your stress!

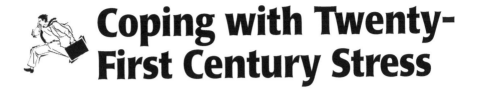

CHAPTER 3

Coping with Twenty-First Century Stress

> ## In This Chapter
>
> ➤ Protecting your personal time
>
> ➤ Pluses and minuses of wireless devices
>
> ➤ Stepping out of the daily grind and learning to relax
>
> ➤ Benefits of vacations

In this chapter, you'll discover how twenty-first century stress can stampede over your life. You'll examine the pace you keep and your relationship with intrusive electronic devices. You'll learn why the American vacation is practically extinct. Plus, you'll find out how to relax and take time out from your fast-paced world and how to cope without getting swallowed up in it.

The Twenty-First Century Culture of Stress

While driving, Sam talks to real estate customers on his smartphone, reads contracts at stoplights, and wolfs down coffee and a bagel for breakfast. Lauren drives her kids to and from school and works a demanding part-time job on her laptop on her kitchen table. Dinner in the oven, one hand on the keyboard, cell phone braced under her chin, she consoles the crying baby she's bouncing on her knee.

Could this be you? Do you hit the ground running the moment your feet touch the floor, checking your iPhone, bolting out the door, chugging a cup of coffee, racing to work with a million thoughts swirling in your head? Are you awash in a sea of errands, a whirlwind of appointments and meetings, trying to keep your head above water, constantly struggling against the limits of time?

Recharging Your Batteries

Finding quiet in the noise and chaos of the twenty-first century is tricky but essential for mastering stress. Studies show that stepping back from your familiar environment gives you new perspectives on your everyday life. When you're bound up in daily stress, it's hard to untangle yourself and see your stressors clearly. Stepping back from the rat race gives you an outsider's view on new ways to handle stress.

There are lots of ways to do this. Trips to new places give you a different environment with which to compare your own life. If you can't travel, you can "get away" by immersing yourself in meditation, prayer, watching nature, a good book, hot bath, or fun craft. Short walks or stretching for a few minutes can help you unwind and clear your head.

Invasion of the Balance Snatchers

Perhaps you feel like you're on a tightrope, trying to hold that line between calm and frantic activity, balancing crammed schedules and clever work gadgets that infiltrate your personal time. The evaporation of personal time can spin you into autopilot, a blur of constant doing, eclipsing your ability to just be, raising stress levels and pulling you further away from yourself and the people you care about.

There was a time when Blackberries were something you consumed, not something that consumed you. And when you had a Bluetooth, you went to the dentist, not to a conference call. The phrase *24/7*, household slang of the twenty-first century, has replaced the *9 to 5* dinosaur adage of the 1990s. These trends indicate how technology has slithered its way into every hour of the day, throwing life off kilter.

Signs of the times: Flextime, twenty-four-hour Walmarts, and wireless leashes—iPads, Blackberries, Androids, Playbooks, iPods, Kindles, laptops, cell phones, Wi-Fi, PDAs, and pagers—all have vaporized the line that once kept *hurry* and *harried* from engulfing the sacred hours of Shabbat, Sunday, and the family dinner hour.

Whether you're a bus driver, factory worker, grocery store clerk, teacher, stay-at-home parent, or president of your own company, listen up. Stress is a huge part of twenty-first-century living. And there's no escaping the frantic pace, time urgency, and lightning speed that pressure you to respond in kind. But as you read on, you'll see that there's a lot you can do to manage and excel at this breakneck pace without breaking your neck.

Multitasking Isn't What It's Cracked Up to Be

Modern life almost makes it necessary for you to be a multitasker to get everything done. And you might consider multitasking to be an essential survival tool in a culture that expects you to change tires going 80 miles an hour. But scientists say that's a bad practice.

While you might think that multitasking is the ticket to more productivity, experts disagree. They say that juggling e-mails, phone calls, and text messages actually undermine your ability to focus and produce. And it fatigues your brain.

Truth Serum

University of Michigan researchers say when you're multitasking, bouncing between several tasks, you're actually forcing your brain to keep refocusing with each rebound and reducing productivity by up to 40 percent. They conclude that multitasking undermines productivity, efficiency, and quality of life by creating several half-baked projects that leave people overwhelmed and stressed out.

Studies from Stanford University confirm that heavy multitaskers have more stress because of trouble focusing and shutting out irrelevant information. In an effort to handle the overload from prolonged multitasking, scientists say, your brain rewires, causing fractured thinking and lack of concentration. As a result, multitaskers take longer to switch among tasks and are less efficient at juggling problems than non-multitaskers.

Tips to Prevent Multitasking from Fatiguing Your Brain

We all have to perform more than one activity at a time once in a while. Here are some tips to help you put the brakes on the frequency of multitasking, remain productive, and prevent you from frying your brain:

➤ Avoid letting your e-mail ping interrupt you during a task. You'll keep your stress level down.

➤ Engage in fewer tasks at one time, and slow down your pace. You'll be more efficient.

➤ Prioritize the most important tasks and finish one big project before revving up another. You won't get overwhelmed.

➤ Keep your mind from jumping to another task by writing it down so you won't forget it, and return to it after you complete your current project. You'll have better focus and concentration.

➤ Bring your attention to the present moment once in a while, notice what's around you, and breathe. You'll be less stressed and more productive in the long run.

Electronic Devices: The New American Idol

The famous Johnny Cash song "I Walk the Line" refers to refraining from love affairs:

I keep a close watch on this heart of mine / I keep my eyes wide open all the time.

But millions of Americans, wedded to their wireless technology, are unable to walk the line. If someone asks you what you think of your iPad or smartphone, you'd probably say you couldn't live without it because it makes your life easier. Most people are so attached to their electronic devices that it's hard to tell who's the master and who's the slave; it's like that old joke when your dog pulls you around on the leash: Are you walking your dog or is your dog walking you?

Trending Now from the Smart Files

➤ A 2011 National Sleep Foundation study reported that 95 percent of people they surveyed use some type of electronic device within an hour of bedtime, which interferes with sleep, at least a few nights a week.

➤ Studies show that 40 percent of workers are interrupted by wireless messages six or more times an hour, while another 37 percent are interrupted three to five times an hour.

➤ A study by the Case Western Reserve School of Medicine reports a link between poor health caused by such behaviors as smoking, drinking, and sexual activity to hyper-texting and hyper-networking.

The Double-Edged Sword of Social Networking

Social networking has revolutionized cultures in the United States and around the world. You might say it has reduced stress, and there's an argument for that. But you could also argue that the Internet has raised stress levels, too.

There's no denying that social networking has helped mitigate stress on a global level. In 2011, Google and Facebook played major roles in helping locate survivors of the earthquake in Japan. Plus, during government unrest in North Africa, Facebook is credited with helping the people of Tunisia and Egypt organize and oust their dictators.

On a personal level, wireless devices save you time. Plus, they are convenient and effective. Imaging studies show the brains of Internet users, for example, are more efficient at finding information. And avid video gamers develop better visual acuity and quicker reaction time than nonplayers.

You can bend over your Kindle at the seashore or coffee shop and read a good book. You can twitter a friend in the Amazon Jungle from your kitchen table or shoot an e-mail to your office in Atlanta from a ski lift in Utah. You can surf the Internet for almost anything you need to find, shop online, and conduct business conferences.

And you can't deny the safety features of electronic gadgets. Instant messaging lets you keep tabs on your home-alone kids while you're miles away in your office. Cell phones help law enforcement locate people in peril. And many of my colleagues conduct therapy sessions over Skype with clients miles away.

The Downside of a Plugged-In Life

"I was itching like a crackhead because I could not use my phone." That comment from a college student participating in a global study conducted by the International Center for Media and the Public Agenda. Researchers asked 1,000 young adults from the United States to Hong Kong to give up all social media for twenty-four hours. When they were deprived of their MP3 players, cell phones, and laptops, stress went through the roof. They experienced elevated heart rates, increased anxiety, panic, irritability, restlessness, and depression. And some say they lost their identity.

In other studies, people confess they have trouble unplugging from electronics because they crave the stimulation. When their device rings, they say they can't resist the urge to answer it. Others admit they get so distracted that they forget dinner plans and family obligations such as picking up the children and become impatient with slower-paced children.

Do Your Wireless Leashes Have a Choke Hold on You?

Take the quiz in Appendix A to see if you are joined at the hip with your electronic devices.

Truth Serum

Experts say that Americans today are more socially isolated because of their love affairs with the Internet, text messages, blogs, Twitter, e-mail, and Facebook. Studies report a one-third drop in the number of people the average American calls a friend. And scientists report that trading sleep, exercise, and relationships for sitting down with electronic gadgets is creating more stress and poor physical and emotional health around the world.

Tips to Spit Shine Your Electronic Habits

Ironically, modern technology is a mixed bag. While relieving you of stress on the one hand, the very electronic gadgets that save time, lives, and improve the quality of life can increase your stress if not properly managed. Allowing wireless intrusions to call the shots automatically puts you in a foot race that'll leave you frazzled. If you didn't pass the test in Appendix A, don't fret. This section has tips that can help you raise your score.

Shock Absorber

Are you just a click away from addiction? As electronics continue to invade private space, you face the challenge of keeping a close watch on your personal life, moving at a reasonable pace, and staying connected to other people in a compassionate, human way. Can you unplug long enough to enjoy life's other pleasures, or do your wireless electronics keep you leashed 24/7? Think of them the way you would a romantic partner. Yes, it's great having them around much of the time. But it's also nice to get a break once in a while, too.

Stay Calm

Stop trying to match the electronic speed of light. The lightning speed of e-mail and cell phones can activate your stress response, provoking a cortisol/dopamine squirt. Then you respond to the immediacy of the device as if it's a threat to extinguish. Slow yourself down and give yourself extra time to get to appointments so you're not always rushing.

Unplug

Manage your devices instead of letting them manage you. Turn off your electronics on breaks, at lunch, and after hours. Carve out blocks of time to work on projects. And don't be duped by the red alert chime of your devices when they interrupt your train of thought. Use custom ring tones for your family, friends, or coworkers when you want to screen calls during off-hours.

At home, put your iPad, cell phone, and pager out of eyesight, just as you would carpentry tools after working on a cabinet in the den. If you must use your wireless devices during personal hours, confine them to specific areas of your home. No work tools in bed, at the table, or in the den while watching TV.

Put the Kibosh on Immediate Checking

Limit the number of times a day you check your e-mail or cell phone to every several hours instead of intermittently. And ease up on instant messaging so you don't create the expectation that you're available 24/7.

Come Up for Air

Take frequent breaks from your wireless devices. Stay in the present with frequent solitary walks to help you unwind and clear your head. Scientists say that stretching and deep breathing release tension, revitalize energy, and refresh a fatigued brain. Experts also advise a fifteen-minute midday power nap to refresh you for the rest of the day.

Block Off Time for Relationships

Think twice before interrupting a face-to-face conversation by answering your Android or BlackBerry. Studies show that wireless intrusions ruin conversational rapport and can damage relationships. Leave space in your schedule for heart-to-heart talks and light-hearted banter with those you care about.

Keep the Rituals in Your Life

Keep the rituals in your life. Studies show that people who celebrate anniversaries, holidays, birthdays, and other important milestones are happier and healthier. On days off, liberate yourself from your wireless leash. Hang out and have fun with friends and family.

Why Relaxing is Hard Work

Bill Zonder is a corporate attorney who refuses to take vacations because he can't be without his smartphone. He's in constant contact with his New York office at lunch, at dinner with his family, and on his fishing boat in the Adirondacks. Unable to disconnect from his wireless devices during downtimes, Bill returns from vacation more stressed out than he was before he left.

What about you? Are you one of the overworked Americans, whose lives are filled with hurrying and rushing, piling on more and more commitments, pressuring yourself with unrealistic deadlines? Do you wail at the clock or drum your fingers when things don't move fast enough? Are you haunted by a sense of time urgency when people don't match your hurried pace? Do you white-knuckle it when you're kept waiting or shun wait lists and waiting rooms as if Dracula is after your blood?

If this description fits you, you could have difficulty relaxing and doing nothing on the beach. Withdrawing from stress is similar to withdrawing from steroids; it creates irritability, restlessness, and agitation. For some people, staying busy mitigates anxiety. If you're one of them and are trying to relax on a beach, you might have trouble keeping stress from bubbling up.

Recharging Your Batteries

Next time you have to wait in rush-hour traffic or a slow-moving line, try calming yourself by accepting the situation exactly as it is. Be willing to kill time even if you hadn't planned to. Tell yourself you're choosing this time to wait so that you're empowered, instead of victimized, by the situation. Bring your attention to the present moment. Stretch and breathe deeply, connecting with the rise and fall of your breath. Then take a quick body scan. Start at your feet and work your way up to your head, relaxing the parts of your body where you feel tension. Instead of getting annoyed when people move at a snail's pace, see them as role models for how you can slow down. Look for mirrors of your own impatience and irritability on the faces of others. Time is never lost when you "choose it and use it" to your advantage, no matter what speed things are moving around you.

The No-Vacation Nation

One of your best antidotes to stress is to take breaks, time off, and vacations. But that's not happening much nowadays. More and more people say they find it hard to relax. And only 57 percent of Americans take their earned vacations.

Why the slow evaporation of the vacation? American employees haul tons of work on leisure trips or refuse vacations altogether because they say extra work responsibilities make it too stressful to take vacations. A common refrain is, "I have to get ahead of my workload in order to leave and then I have to work doubly hard when I get back, and I'm worried the whole time because I'm getting behind. It's not worth the stress."

Others say they're afraid they'll be perceived as a slacker, get passed over for job promotions, or that someone might be angling for their job. Still others are so plugged into laptops, cell phones, and BlackBerrys that they come back from vacation more exhausted than they were when they left.

Trending Now from the Smart Files

Here are some statistics on the vanishing American vacation:

➤ In 2010, 37 percent of working Americans didn't take all their vacation days, up from 34 percent in 2009.

➤ 55 percent of working Americans say they come back from time off still not rested and rejuvenated after vacation.

➤ 50 percent of US executives say they don't use all of their earned vacation because it's too stressful to take time off.

Take a Vacation Instead of a Guilt Trip

Do you feel guilty taking time off when there's so much work to be done? If it's hard for you to relax, here are some steps you can take to go on guilt-free vacations and even enjoy them:

➤ Set boundaries: There is something to be said for preventive stress. Limited communication with the office while vacationing can be less stressful than worrying about things piling up. Feeling that you're getting behind can make you feel out of control and more stressed. Strictly enforced limits on vacation such as an hour a day to check e-mail or make phone calls are important if you want to relax.

➤ Buffer your work exits and reentries: Don't work right up until the moment you leave and head back to work right off the plane. If possible, schedule an extra day off before you depart and another when you come back to ease back in.

➤ Balance activities: Alternate your time between staying active and resting. A walk on the beach combined with ten minutes of meditation both give you a biochemical boost. Activity raises endorphins. Quieting your mind stimulates the part of your brain that dampens the surges of adrenaline and cortisol accompanying stress.

➤ Plan ahead: Choose a person you trust to manage day-to-day tasks during your absence, and make sure your coworkers know you'll be away. Designate a point person to be contacted on your voice mail and out-of-office e-mail only on matters you want to be bothered about.

➤ Work at not working: Ask yourself, "Why do I work this way? Why am I rushing through life?" Some people have a habit of judging themselves. If you believe what you do is never enough, it can make you pile on more stress. Examine your own tendencies to create stress for yourself. It might lead you to insight.

Take a "Staycation"

If it's too stressful to catch a plane or travel long distances by car, consider vacationing at home. But if you take a staycation, make sure you unplug from your usual routines. It's important to spend your time engaged in different activities around the house that you enjoy but never get to do, such as gardening or a special hobby. Or take a day trip to a fun place where you've been itching to go but haven't had time.

"Rx from Dr. Bryan"

The Doctor Of Calm Is In

Vacation is what you take when you can't take what you've been taking any longer.

—*The Cowardly Lion in* The Wizard of Oz

My prescription: Vacations are like prescriptions for what ails you. The whole point of vacations is to restore your mind and body and get a new lease on life. If you can take a vacation and leave work, worry, and problems behind, my hat is off to you. If you can't, find a way to unplug from the office and your work tools now and then. Escape into a vacation, staycation, or playcation even if it's just for a day or even a few hours, just for the health of it! Here's to outsmarting your stress!

CHAPTER 4

Preventing Burnout and Creating a Stress-Free Life

In This Chapter

➤ Signs of burnout

➤ Preventing burnout

➤ Healthy stress management

➤ Your perspective on stress

In this chapter, you'll discover how stress can cause burnout and how you can prevent it. You'll examine unhealthy ways people cope with stress and gain healthy strategies for stress mastery. Plus, you'll get tips on how to prevent your perspective from contributing to your stress level and how to use it to your advantage.

Putting Teeth into Stress Proofing

Constantly snowed under at work? Behind the eight ball as bills pile up? When you're facing stress, you cope in the best way you know how. Usually that means relying on your street sense—the resources you've learned from life—and your perspective of the situation. But sometimes that's not enough to stress proof your life, especially if you've had a checkered stress history. You could still be mopping up from your last stress hit. So let's put some teeth into preventing burnout and creating a stress-free life.

Dodging Burnout

How well you master stress and fend off burnout depends on several factors: the degree to which you take care of yourself, coping skills developed over time, and your perspective on stress. Let's start with defining *burnout*.

In the still-lonely hours before dawn, Sara Martin plops in her armchair, grabs a fistful of hair, and stares out the window at the black sky—hopeless thoughts racing, heart pounding. Another sleepless night with her mortgage past due, and she just got laid off from her job. Once debt-free after sacrificing her personal life for a position at the top of the company's career ladder, now Sara has lost her spark. Worn down and worn out, she sighs, "I have nothing left to give." Sara is burned out—she is one of many people who cave when pressures get to be too much and everything seems to fall apart like a house of cards.

What Is Burnout?

The buzzword *burnout* was coined by Herbert Freudenberger in 1974. To this day, burnout is not recognized as a legitimate psychological or psychiatric disorder. But it is a condition linked to depression, anxiety, and stress-related illnesses that receives a lot of attention from the helping professions and people dealing with situational pressures.

Stress is one thing; burnout is a completely different state of mind. Under stress, you still struggle to cope with pressures. But once burnout takes hold, you're out of gas and you've given up all hope of surmounting your obstacles. When you're suffering from burnout, it's more than just fatigue. There's a deep sense of disillusionment and hopelessness that your efforts have been in vain. Life loses its meaning, and small tasks feel like a hike up Mount Everest. Your interests and motivation dry up, and you fail to meet your obligations.

Stress Vocab

Burnout is a state of physical and mental exhaustion over disappointment brought about by prolonged stress and dedication to a job, a cause, a way of life, or a relationship that failed to produce the expected outcome.

No one is immune to burnout. It can hit the high-achieving executive who feels overworked and undervalued, the nurse or clergyperson in a caregiving role around the clock, or the stay-at-home mom who juggles childrearing, carpooling, housework, and a teetering marriage. But the biggest source of burnout is in the work arena, where Americans are burning out at an alarming rate.

Trending Now from the Smart Files

Here are some statistics on burnout in the United States:

➤ According to a 2011 CareerBuilder survey, a whopping 77 percent of workers feel burnout at work and 46 percent say their workloads increased in the last six months.

➤ More than 60 percent of work absenteeism is attributed to psychological stress and stress-related burnout.

➤ More than 40 percent of pastors and 47 percent of their spouses report that they are suffering from spiritual and emotional burnout.

➤ An estimated 25 to 60 percent of physicians say they experience burnout.

Signs of Burnout

There's no stress escape hatch. But you can take a number of actions to identify and prevent burnout. First, it's important to recognize some of the signs of burnout:

➤ Disillusionment/loss of meaning

➤ Mental and physical fatigue

➤ Moodiness, impatience, and short temperedness

➤ Loss of motivation and interest in commitments

➤ Inability to meet obligations

➤ Lowered immunity to illness

➤ Emotional detachment from previous involvements

➤ Feeling efforts are unappreciated

➤ Withdrawal from people and social situations

➤ Hopeless, helpless, and depressed outlook

➤ Job absenteeism and inefficiency

➤ Sleep deprivation

➤ Foggy thinking and trouble concentrating

Compassion Fatigue

The inability to say no and put yourself first takes its toll, especially if you're expected to bring empathy to the suffering of others. Your focus on caring can put you in danger of self-neglect. Over time, self-neglect can lead you to become so mentally and physically depleted that you plunge into compassion fatigue.

Stress Vocab

Compassion fatigue, or compassion burnout, is physical exhaustion and a depletion of emotional energy brought on by the stress of caring for and helping others at the expense of taking care of yourself.

Whether you're caring for an aging parent in your home, overseeing young children, advocating for the needy, or tending to the sick in hospitals, you could be vulnerable. Physicians, nurses, counselors, and the clergy are a few professions that are more susceptible to compassion fatigue. Feelings of exhaustion, frustration, discouragement, and helplessness are a few of the indicators.

Recharging Your Batteries

Fortunately, you can recharge your batteries if you're facing burnout. Once you acknowledge the problem, you can start to say no and practice self-care. A colleague asks you to do something you don't have time to do and you say no. You speak up when a friend takes advantage of your good nature. You refuse to bail a loved one out of trouble for the umpteenth time.

Sometimes the best way to care for others is to self-care by drawing a line that protects you from stress. So develop a healthy attitude about what's humanly possible for you. Tell yourself there's a limit, and put the rest out of the picture. Think of this attitude as a sign of strength, not weakness. Remember: caring and detachment are twins, not enemies.

Is Stress Making You Old Before Your Time?

You know your birthday, but do you know your stress age? The stress you're under could be making you old before your time. A frazzled lifestyle combined with your perception of stress and your unique way of dealing with it create chemical changes in your body. Impatience, procrastination, anger, and need to control are just a few personality traits that contribute to your stress. I'll discuss the relationship between personality traits and stress in detail in Chapter 5.

The wear and tear of stress and the way you deal with it can make your mind and body older or younger than you think. Appendix A provides a simple test that gives you a thumbnail sketch of how stress and the cortisol juices you stew in could be affecting your health, even taking years off your life.

After taking the test, if you find that stress is making you older than you are, you don't have to retire to your bed and pull the covers over your head. Look back over the twenty questions. Identify stressful habits that you could change to develop a healthier lifestyle to keep you from getting old before your time. Hold tight. As you continue reading, you'll discover ways to add back years to your life and make it richer and more satisfying.

Unhealthy Ways of Managing Stress

You don't have to wait around for stress to slug you. By now, you recognize the telltale signs and sources of your stress. The next step is to take charge of it in small, manageable ways before it grabs hold of you. If you're like many people, you've resorted to unhealthy strategies to handle stress, some of which can cause quicker burnout. After you have a clearer picture of what you've been doing, I'll give you some tips on healthy ways to manage stress. Replacing unhealthy strategies with healthier techniques can help you cope with pressures and dodge burnout.

Quick Relief versus Long-Term Health

Notice some of the old ways you've handled stress that haven't worked for you, such as avoiding something stressful by sleeping or watching TV, or smoking, drinking, or eating too much. Unfortunately, most people develop bad habits to cope with stress. And, if you're anything like them, you're not thinking about your health, either; you're thinking about quick relief.

Bad Habits that Don't Work

The American Psychological Association did a breakdown of the unhealthy ways Americans manage stress in a pinch. From its list below, see if any of the bad habits ring a bell with you or if you've developed others that you can add to the list?

➤ Overeating or eating unhealthy foods: 48 percent

➤ Skipping meals: 39 percent

➤ Napping: 43 percent women, 32 percent men

➤ Shopping: 25 percent women, 11 percent men

➤ Drinking alcohol: 18 percent

➤ Smoking: 16 percent

Shock Absorber

Step off the stress roller coaster and soften your landing. Make your personal care a top priority with stress cushions. The more you cushion yourself from daily stress, the more you have to give to others. Exercise that you enjoy, tasty nutritious food, and a good night's sleep are the trifecta for a calm, stress-free life. All three basics are keys to regulating your body's stress level and keeping your energy up and health problems down. And as you practice setting limits on the demands placed upon you, leave elbow room to stretch, breathe, meditate, look out the window, or take a trek around the block.

Healthy Strategies for Managing Stress

In order to minimize stress, you need to make sure you choose healthy strategies for dealing with it. There are some actions you can take right off the bat to reduce your stress. As you practice these tips, you'll discover that you're more efficient at what you do.

Check Your Attitude

Start with your attitude. Think of any changes you make as self-care instead of self-deprivation. You'll have more luck managing stress if you think of daily exercise as a healthy investment instead of physical drudgery. Or think of foregoing that extra piece of cake or glass of wine as nurturing instead of punishing yourself.

Plan something to look forward to. Substitute worry and stressful thoughts with your positive plans. Simple new thoughts such as inviting someone you enjoy for dinner or taking a short trip to see a loved one can make you feel more in charge of your stress.

Focus on What You Can Control

Make two columns. Under the first one, list all the stressors you can't control such as the weather and traffic. In the second column, list all the things you can control such as your outlook. Then, focus on making improvements to the items in the second column one by one and one step at a time.

Step Out of Your Stress Rut

Choose one thing to do differently, no matter how small. In a way, it doesn't matter what it is as long as you interrupt your stress paralysis. Stop stewing in your cortisol juices. Get off the couch and walk around the block, take a different route home from the office, invite a new coworker to lunch, or face a challenge that's frightened you. In small ways you're sending yourself a huge signal: "I'm in charge, and I'm doing something about it."

Make Tradeoffs

Motivate yourself to develop healthier new habits. Do the things you like best only after you've added one healthy thing you've put off or dreaded doing. Let's say you love surfing the Internet or going on Facebook. You make a deal with yourself that you have to earn every hour you spend on the Internet with a half hour of physical activity first.

Recharging Your Batteries

Simon and Garfunkel said it best:

Slow down, you move too fast / you've got to make the morning last.

Take a deep breath, step back from your life, and reset your pace, making elbow room for downtime. Even if it's only five minutes, downtime can help you quiet your mind, put the brakes on your stress response, and activate your calm response. Make a conscious effort to turn off your battery. Then slow down, kick back, and treat yourself like a human being instead of a machine. Studies show that moving at a steady pace puts you at the finish line before frantic racing against the clock. Plus, you get to enjoy life as it's happening, instead of rushing through it and going down in flames. After all, the turtle won the race.

Pamper Yourself

Indulge yourself in healthy activities that you enjoy and that quiet your mind and relax your body. Here are a few suggestions:

- ➤ Read a book
- ➤ Watch a movie
- ➤ Listen to soft music
- ➤ Soak in a hot bath
- ➤ Get a massage, manicure, facial, or pedicure
- ➤ Take a yoga or meditation class
- ➤ Develop a fun hobby

Develop a Support Network

When you have a strong support network, you do a better job of managing stress. If you're under stress, avoid isolating yourself. Make sure you have connections with people who respect and support you. Stay in touch with friends and loved ones, especially when pressures mount. Social contacts give you a place to air your tensions instead of keeping them bottled up so that stress doesn't isolate you.

Your Perspective on Stress

At first, you might think there's nothing you can do about your stress. Some stress comes from life circumstances and some you create yourself. As you think about your own stress pattern, notice how much comes from outside of you and how much from within you. You'll start to see that you have more control than you think. Sometimes you can turn a situation around; sometimes you can prevent stress by changing your course of action. But much of the time changing your outlook is the most powerful de-stressor in your toolbox.

Ask Not How Stress Is Treating You; Ask How You Are Treating Stress

It's true: your relationships will always have challenges, the bills aren't going to stop coming, people will continue to disappoint you, there will never be twenty-five hours in your day to get everything done, you won't succeed at everything you attempt, and you're going to get sick from time to time. And these are stressful situations. But you can't blame life, the job, relationships, kids, the weather, traffic, or any other outside factors for *all* of your stress.

It helps to ask yourself if you're somehow adding to your stress without realizing it. When you take a breath and step back from your life, you might be surprised by how much of your stress comes from your perspective. It can be a real eye-opener to ask yourself how you're treating stress, instead of what stress is doing to you. This strategy helps you see yourself as being in charge and pressing outward against the stress instead of stress pressing inward upon you, holding you prisoner. This can be the start to a clearer picture of where your stress comes from.

Truth Serum

Your stress level is a consequence of the situation you're in combined with the view you take of it. Your heart races before a competitive tennis match the same as it does before you confront your boss. But you label tennis as fun and facing your boss as stress. If you evaluate an event as a problem, then you'll experience stress. If you label it as an adventure, you'll feel excitement. For some people, ziplining is stressful; for me, it's an adventure. For me, bungee jumping is stressful; for some people, it's an adventure.

You can even set off your stress response by just imagining yourself in a negative situation such as having a disagreement with your boss. When you develop a habit of creating stress in your head, it takes its toll. But you can reverse the process by paying attention to how you're looking at stressful situations. Take a bird's-eye view, and see if there's anything about your perspective you can change. It might make some things you thought were insurmountable feel like a breeze.

Psst, Look Right in Front of You

If you're like most people, when you're under stress, you don't realize it. Sometimes taking charge of your stress is like the little lady looking for her glasses when they're on her nose the whole time. It's easy to overlook ways that you contribute to your stress because you've been doing things a certain way for so long. But when you take a hard look at your own habits, routines, excuses, and attitudes, you will find more clarity in identifying your true sources of stress. Here are some examples:

➤ You've blamed your stress on a demanding job, but when you take a closer look, you discover that it's your inability to say no that causes you to be overloaded.

➤ Worry over meeting a deadline overwhelms you because of your procrastination instead of the deadline itself.

➤ You know you're frustrated that your career hasn't been as successful as you'd dreamed. But could it be that your fear of sticking your neck out—rather than your boss, the job, or more successful coworkers—holds you back?

➤ You're aware that you constantly fret about not having enough money to pay the monthly bills. Maybe overspending, instead of mounting bills, causes the financial stress.

Discover What's Underneath Your Stress

To discover what's underneath your stress, follow the steps in this formula to see if you've overlooked the real source:

I know I'm stressed out/worried about_____. But maybe it's_____ instead of_____ that's causing my stress. I can take charge of this stressor by_____.

1. Start with what you know to be a stressor: I know I'm stressed out about being snowed under at work.

2. Then, ask yourself if you've overlooked a habit or attitude, and plug that possibility into the formula: But maybe it's because my perfectionism makes it hard for me to share the load.

3. Instead of what you thought it was: Instead of job pressures, my drive to take on more work is what's causing my stress.

4. I can take charge of this stressor by: delegating more at work or saying no to a request when I'm already overloaded.

5. Summarize your findings in your stress journal.

Shock Absorber

Do some soul searching on your stress perspective. Check in with yourself periodically but always with compassion. If you're constantly arguing with family members or squabbling with coworkers, you might gently ask yourself, "Where's the common denominator?" Could your stress come from forcing your way of doing things or resisting someone else's point of view? Suppose you've sunk into a worry rut as a coping mechanism, not realizing that it doesn't help and only makes matters worse. Or you might've gotten into a habit of negative thinking that causes you to see the glass as half empty instead of half full. After you've looked closer at stressful situations, ask yourself what, if anything, you can do to reduce stress and create more harmony in your life.

Get a Reality Check

It's easy to lock yourself into one way of viewing a stressful event. Getting a reality check from a friend, family member, or support group and comparing their perspectives to yours can help you manage stressful situations. For example, you might read an irritating tone into your boss's voice mail. The feedback from a friend who listens to it might give you a different perspective, lowering your stress.

If all else fails, try a support group, even if it's an informal group of friends or a network of professionals. In severe stress cases, where adequate support is unavailable, you might need to seek professional help to assess the need for medication and/or learn healthy coping skills and stress management.

How Do You Stack Up?

If you were to make a list from most to least of the important people and activities in your life, where would you fall? Would you even make the list? If so, how far down the list would you be? If you put yourself at the bottom and stack your tasks on top, you risk burnout.

Ask yourself if you're putting everybody else's needs at the top of the list and yours last. Self-sacrifice is a noble act, so we are told. But when you put yourself at the bottom of the heap, stress and burnout deplete what you could give to your job, loved ones, and friends.

"Rx from Dr. Bryan"

The Doctor Of Calm Is In

Self-love is not so vile a sin as self-neglecting

—William Shakespeare

When you take care of yourself first—making sure you get the right amount of rest, exercise, and nutrition and that you do things that interest and replenish you—there's more of you to go around. My prescription: Take one dose of self-care first thing in the morning and one before bedtime. Refills indefinite. Here's to outsmarting your stress!

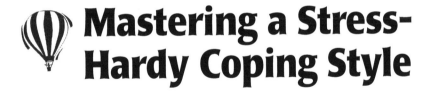 Mastering a Stress-Hardy Coping Style

In This Chapter

> ➤ Stress coping styles
>
> ➤ A well-balanced coping style
>
> ➤ What stress hardiness is
>
> ➤ Cultivating stress hardiness

In this chapter, you'll learn how some personality types actually increase stress while trying to reduce it. You'll find out why some people cave and others thrive under stress. And you'll pinpoint where you fall on the scale. Plus, you'll discover the qualities it takes to achieve balance and gain tips on how to develop stress resilience.

Your Stress Coping Style

As you may know by now, each of us responds to high-pressured situations in different ways. Some people get energized, ratchet up their inner resources, and thrive. Others muddle through or succumb to stress, watching their dreams blow up in smoke.

Are you the type who tackles stress head-on or do you retreat? In balance, each approach has value. But in the extreme, both can be self-defeating and create more stress. Studies show that although there's no one-size-fits-all approach, the best path to stress resilience is to find balance at a point in between the extremes.

By nature, everybody has a predominant style of coping with stress. And you're about to discover yours. Some people have a self-defeating approach that raises rather than lowers their stress temperature. Stress vigilantes go overboard in their attempts to control stress. They have difficulty backing off or letting go. At the other extreme, stress avoiders have trouble stepping up to the plate and facing their stressors. Let's see where you fall.

Recharging Your Batteries

Understanding your stress coping style helps you pinpoint habits you can change to develop stress resilience. If you're a stress vigilante striving for balance, you need to loosen up and let go more. You need a certain amount of worry and control to keep you safe, but too much or too little creates more harm than good. If you're a stress avoider, you find balance with more direct action. You can develop fearlessness, step up to the plate, and face the stressors that have gotten a free pass. There are times when you need to slack off and appease. But in the extreme, these traits backfire, raising your stress temperature. The trick is to learn to worry or control well and to slack off and appease well, at the right time, to the right degree.

Stress Vigilantes

Forethought, preparation, and planning are qualities that arm you with good stress-prevention strategies. But if you go too far, you might fall into the category of stress vigilantes—people who go overboard, overreacting to the possibilities of stress. If you're a stress vigilante, you attack stress with all guns blazing, anticipating and controlling situations. In trying to preempt stress, you actually create more of it with your extreme approach. Examples of stress vigilantes are the control freak, the crisis junkie, the perfectionist, the careaholic, and the worry wart.

The Control Freak

Your controlling nature makes it hard for you to share the load or to work as a team member. You believe no one can do the job as well as you can, and that asking for help is a sign of weakness. You tend to overplan and overorganize so that conditions are predictable, consistent, and controllable. When you overload, overwhelm, and isolate yourself, it dampens your spontaneity and flexibility. To bring balance, learn to delegate and prioritize. Be more flexible and spontaneous and be willing to work with others.

The Crisis Junkie

In an attempt to eliminate stress, you're impatient and in a hurry to get tasks completed. But because nothing moves fast enough for you, your impatience creates more stress and more crises. The more items you can cross off your list, the better you feel. A job left hanging is out of the question. Your preference to engage in several activities at once gives you a false sense of accomplishment. You despise waiting and try almost anything to get to the front of the line. Your snap decisions cause you to make avoidable mistakes that take additional time to repair. To bring balance, learn to relax and wait. Take a calmer approach and do one thing at a time.

The Perfectionist

Your standards for yourself and others are unattainable, leaving no room for mistakes. In your attempt to eliminate stress, you judge yourself (and others) unmercifully, trying to cover all the bases and get it right. But you end up overloading yourself so that you don't have time for your own needs. Your stress level goes through the roof from the inhuman burdens you place on yourself. Feelings of failure, anger at others, and burnout are constant companions. Change requires a basic shift in attitude. To bring balance, do your best but give yourself elbow room to make mistakes and learn from them.

The Careaholic

You're on a mission to rescue people even if they don't need it. Overloading yourself with other people's problems is a distraction from your own. If you're focused on helping someone else, you don't have to think of your own burdens. While being in service to others keeps the focus off you, your world is crumbling under your feet. And you risk compassion burnout. To regain balance, examine your own unmet needs that you've avoided with your careaholism. Then take care of yourself first before taking on the burdens of others .

The Worry Wart

You're an excessive worrier. Although most of what plagues you never happens, you go through the stress of it anyway, and you risk physical illness. Constant worry is an attempt to predict the future and prepare for an unknown outcome. To bring balance, eliminate as many problems as you can. Then accept and make the best of what you can't control. Remember that worry cannot predict the future. It doesn't prepare you for anything, so don't give it your power. Calm your worried mind with some of the relaxation techniques such as yoga, changing your perspective, meditation, and deep breathing that I discuss in later chapters.

Truth Serum

People with type A personalities, are hard-driven, competitive, hurried, and can be hostile. They are compulsive overachievers who try to accomplish more and more in less time. By nature, type As have many traits of stress vigilantes. They are constantly busy with several tasks at once, move at a rapid pace, halfheartedly pay attention to conversations, and are unable to sit for long periods. As type As reach for the stars, they ignore fatigue and physical aches and pains that warn of stress-related health problems. They risk burnout, coronary artery and heart disease, and other illnesses. If you or someone you know is Type A, don't fret. You can modify your stress coping skills with proper diet, regular exercise, and ample sleep. Plus, you can slow down your pace, limit tasks, do one thing at a time, and stay in the present moment.

Stress Avoiders

Sometimes avoidance is a good way to manage stress. But for situations that require attention, too much avoidance creates stress. If you're a stress avoider, stalling, delaying, or retreating might seem like the best way to handle stress. But in the extreme, this self-defeating coping strategy gives stress a free pass to stampede your life. Examples of stress avoiders are the procrastinator, the appeaser, the sad sack, and the slacker.

The Procrastinator

Because procrastination often is based in fear, putting off preparing for stressful events gives temporary relief. You don't have to deal with the immediate fear of failing. But stalling makes matters worse. It adds a second layer of pressure, throwing you into a stress cycle. Suppose you put off preparing for a job interview because thinking about it stresses you out. Dragging it out raises your tension level and lets things pile up, overwhelming you even more. To bring balance, face your stressors head-on and early instead of waiting until the last minute. When you have several items on your list, start with the ones you can accomplish quickly to help you get motivated.

The Appeaser

Winston Churchill said it best: "An appeaser is one who feeds a crocodile, hoping it will eat him last." You are afraid of disapproval. So you avoid conflict by agreeing with people even when you don't agree. Pleasing people puts you under pressure to keep up a façade, and you end up turning yourself into a pretzel to gain approval. But being appeasing has a short shelf life. No matter how hard you try, someone will disapprove of something—and it's only a matter of time before the crocodile will feast upon you. To regain balance, take a stand, learn to disagree or say no instead of yes. Be your own person, gauge your actions by your own standards, not by the opinions of others.

The Sad Sack

You see yourself as a helpless pawn of fate. You believe you have no say-so over what happens to you, that your life is determined by external circumstances. You're afraid to take chances or try new avenues to face stress because you believe your actions won't make a difference. Instead of trying to manage everyday pressures, you give up and become a victim of them. You approach life with self-pity and sadness, blaming other people and situations for your plight. To bring balance, take more responsibility and be more proactive by facing your stressors. Try new things, stick your neck out, and learn to believe in yourself.

The Slacker

You see the big picture but have trouble with details. You have creative ideas, start many projects, but get bored with the follow-through. You're easily distracted and start new projects before completing the ones underway. You have many half-baked projects and missed deadlines that overwhelm you. You're viewed by others as a slacker who doesn't live up to commitments. To bring balance, learn to focus on details and finish one project before starting another one. When it comes to deadlines, refrain from multitasking and procrastination.

Shock Absorber

Most people have aspects of both the stress vigilante and the stress avoider. In the extreme, either stress style can work against you. Where you fall on the scale depends on several factors: personality traits, upbringing, and situational conditions. Regardless of your makeup, research shows you can change old habits of drowning under pressure and learn to keep your head above water. Determine whether you lean in the direction of stress vigilante or stress avoider, or whether you are a combination of several different types. Then decide what actions you can take to modify certain aspects of your stress style and create more balance in your life. Record the findings in your stress journal.

Stress Hardiness and Stress Sensitivity

You might think that staying away from stress is the best way to manage it. But is it really? It depends on your individual personality. Some people do better avoiding stress, but others thrive on it. Scientists call people who respond well to pressures stress hardy, compared to stress-sensitive people who are shattered by stress.

Stress Vocab

Stress hardiness is the mindset of people who view stressful circumstances as an opportunity, instead of a problem, that allows them to overcome and grow from pressures without avoiding or caving into them.

Truth Serum

Studies show that stress hardiness is present early in life. During the 1980s, social scientists studied the phenomenon of resilient children—those reared in poverty, by schizophrenic parents, or in abusive households. Despite their dire upbringings, these children had an exceptional ability to handle stress, and they thrived in spite of their traumatic circumstances. Early family misfortunes, instead of destroying their motivations, fueled their intellectual and creative potential.

In contrast to vulnerable children who feel helpless, resilient children exercise personal control over their surroundings. As adults, they thrive, becoming high achievers. Do these children sound like the stress-hardy telephone executives to you?

The Origins of Stress Hardiness

The idea of stress hardiness grew from scientists charged with evaluating the psychological well-being of executives under high stress in the 1970s. During the restructuring of a telephone company, researchers identified a group of executives with exceptional personality traits that protected them from the ravages of stress.

During the restructuring, many executives succumbed to stress. Some died of heart attacks, became violent, got divorced, and had overall poor mental health. But one-third of them thrived under the stress. Their health improved, careers soared, and relationships flourished. According to the scientists, the stress-hardy executives had a whopping 50 percent reduction in stress-related health problems compared to managers without stress hardiness.

Are You Stress Sensitive or Stress Hardy?

Today, the notion of stress hardiness has become a road map for how you, too, can let stress roll off your back. Some people are naturally born stress hardy, less affected by stressful situations and more resilient to change. Others are more vulnerable to the arrows of everyday stress.

If you're vulnerable to stress, you believe your life is determined by external forces more powerful than you. You think you have no control over what happens and that it doesn't pay to try hard because things never work out in your favor. You're used to thinking of yourself as downtrodden, and you focus on hardships and problems that keep you stuck. Your chronic feelings of failure, despair, and self-pity leave you wide open to stress.

Extra Sensitivity to Environmental Stressors

It was a humid July Fourth picnic. Luke, a former Marine, wolfed down his grilled burger as the American flag curled in the air and flashbacks of war swirled in his head. The sudden exploding fireworks launched him out of his lawn chair. In that split instant, Luke's post-traumatic stress disorder (PTSD) catapulted him back into combat.

Stress Vocab

Post Traumatic Stress Disorder (PTSD) is an extreme form of stress brought about by a life-threatening event such as combat, a natural disaster, violent crime, serious accident, or physical or sexual abuse.

Long after the traumatic event is over, PTSD continues to take a toll. It makes the person with PTSD feel danger in situations that remind him or her of that event. The person experiences the threat as if it's happening all over again when activated by an environmental event.

In addition to PTSD, several other forms of stress sensitivity result from a biochemical response in the brain to environmental triggers:

➤ If you're what's known as a highly sensitive person (HSP), your thin-skinned stress response is highly tuned to your surroundings and emotionally charged situations.

➤ If you have attention deficit disorder (ADD), you're more sensitive to distractions that interfere with your ability to focus and concentrate on tasks.

➤ If you have seasonal affective disorder (SAD), you have a mood-altering condition that makes you more sensitive to light deprivation and darkness. It can lead to depression and lethargy in winter months when the sun is farther away from the earth.

The good news is that all of these conditions are treatable. With proper professional counseling, medical support, and community resources, you can gain more control over environmental stressors and enjoy life again.

Shock Absorber

Soft heart, a sponge for other people's moods and criticism, choked up by the beauty of a sunset—these are just a few hallmarks of the highly sensitive person (HSP). If you are an HSP, your amplified nervous system allows more of the world to penetrate you, and you experience the world in high definition. You have heightened stress reactions to bright lights, loud noises, scratchy fabrics, sharp colors, large crowds, strong smells, and people's emotions. On the upside, HSPs have compassion for what others are going through and sensitivity to small things. HSPs make up 20 percent of the population. And they are born, not made.

If you wear your heart on your sleeve, try nurturing your overactive stress response. Take measures to buffer your overexcited brain: wear ear plugs to sleep or cushion loud noises and avoid negative people who drain you. Give yourself plenty of refueling time with quiet time, calm moments such as a hot bath, meditation, and massage.

Three Cs of Stress-Hardy People

Studies show that when you see yourself as being a cause instead of an effect in your life, you'll be more optimistic and respond more positively to situations beyond your control. When you're stress hardy, you tend to have three outstanding personality traits:

➤ Control: You believe you have control over events in your life. You're master of your fate and bear responsibility for what happens to you. You know there are situations you cannot control, but you know you can choose how to react. You believe your actions determine positive or negative outcomes. And you know if you make a mistake, instead of caving, you can do something to make it right, that you can affect your tomorrow by how you handle today.

➤ Challenge: You're more optimistic by nature and misfortune fuels your motivation to perform well. You view stress as a challenge instead of a threat and look for opportunities to overcome pressures instead of ways to deny or avoid them. Instead of feeling helpless and debilitated, you welcome situations that offer a chance for you to improve and turn a negative experience into a positive one.

➤ Commitment: You are committed to something bigger than yourself. You take advantage of social support and are deeply involved in your work and relationships. Your curiosity about life moves you outward into new, unknown territory instead of inward into retreat. You don't operate in a vacuum. Your shared struggle with others toughens you, giving a greater cause to your efforts. Your commitment to others, to the common good, and to team spirit trumps your own concerns.

Shock Absorber

If you're a pessimist, you probably take adversity personally, see it as permanent, and believe there's nothing you can do about it. You're more likely than an optimist to succumb to stress under pressure. If you're a true optimist, you roll with the punches. You see adversity as temporary, specific, and external to your life. You don't take hardships personally and believe that you can overcome them. If you lean toward pessimism, try not to take setbacks personally and take a more positive outlook. Later chapters will give you tips on how to cultivate optimism for better stress resilience.

Are You Steel, Plastic, or Glass?

How stress hardy are you? It depends on the way you look at life. To find out, answer yes or no to the questions in the quiz in Appendix A called Are You Steel, Plastic, or Glass?

Tips to Buff Up Your Stress Hardiness

Just as lifting weights develops physical stamina, facing stressors builds inner strength, equipping you to face life's hardships head-on. There are some steps you can take to buff up your stress hardiness.

Face Challenges

Look at adversity as a challenge instead of a threat. Try to find something in the stressful event that you can learn and grow from. Don't wait for disaster to hit. Look at life as an adventure to experience, not a problem to solve. So when challenges hit, you're more equipped to face them, so you don't avoid them. Instead of latching on to the easy life, expose yourself to small challenges that hone your skills for the bigger ones yet to come. You can develop more fearlessness that will serve you in future challenges.

Pump Up Your Internal Control

Ask yourself what you can control in a stressful situation, focus on that, and let the rest go. Internal control comes from finding ways around stressful obstacles instead of falling victim to them. If it's raining, move the party inside. To avoid stressful traffic, leave earlier for work, take public transit, change your attitude, or enjoy soft music when stuck in gridlock. You can't control the economy, but if you're worried about finding a job, you can update your resume, connect with a network, and cast a wide net with your job search. Usually taking action, instead of folding your arms and giving up, empowers you to overcome the challenges.

Seek Support

You have more stress hardiness when you know someone has your back. Your bonds with friends and loved ones anchor you from instability and help you cultivate inner strength. When you have supporters on your side, it gives you the "social capital" to jump-start your motivation. If you get discouraged and feel like giving up, knowing that others are counting on you keeps your spirit alive. Feeling part of a group with an obligation to more than yourself can build your determination.

Shock Absorber

People with stress hardiness are not immune to stress. They take their stress hits now and then like the rest of us do. But they're tougher about picking themselves up, brushing themselves off, and facing challenges. If you weren't one of the lucky ones born with stress hardiness, research shows that you can develop it with time and patience. As long as you're willing to practice being more optimistic, flexible, and constructive in your reactions to pressure, you can become strong like steel and watch stress ping off of you.

Get Physically Fit

Studies link physical fitness to stress hardiness. Exercise toughens your body as well as your mind and makes you more resistant to stress. People who exercise regularly notice that they are more tolerant of hassles and minor annoyances such as waiting in lines or traffic snarls. Develop an exercise regimen, preferably an activity you enjoy, that matches your physical abilities, and stick with it.

Avoid Becoming Overwhelmed

Give yourself pep talks and rewards along the way to your goals. Try not to overwhelm yourself by biting off more than you can chew. When something feels too big, break it down and take each task as it comes one step at a time. Instead of sweating the small stuff, ask yourself what's really important and make that a priority. Then, let the rest slide.

Be True to Yourself

Accept your personal limitations while nudging yourself to try new things. Being stress hardy doesn't mean opposing who you truly are at your core. It's about sticking your neck out and doing something you've put off or were afraid to do. Studies show that people who embrace challenges as a natural part of living are less likely to crumble under pressure. So stretch yourself and toughen up, but don't force yourself to become someone you're not.

Befriend Your Stressors

Yes, you heard me right. I realize it sounds counter-intuitive, but forging a friendlier relationship with stress actually can help you reduce your stress level. You might be rolling your eyes right now. But think of stress as your protector, and consider all the ways it takes care of you. It watches out for you when you're driving in heavy traffic, using hazardous materials or equipment, or searching for your car in a dark parking garage. It motivates you to meet deadlines, earn a good grade on a test, and win your boss's confidence with a persuasive argument. In many ways, it's your friend.

"Rx from Dr. Bryan"

The Doctor Of Calm Is In

So whether it's anger or craving or jealousy or fear or depression—whatever it might be—the notion is not to get rid of it, but to make friends with it

—Pema Chodron

My prescription: Set aside time to think about the flip side of stress. Make a list of all the times stress had your back when you thought it was against you. Read over your list once daily before or after meals or until you're calmer and more appreciative. Notice if a change in your perspective reduces your stress and helps you cultivate a calmer, clearer mind. If negative symptoms persist after forty-eight hours, double your daily dosage. Here's to outsmarting your stress!

PART TWO

Adopting a Healthy Lifestyle: The Trifecta of Stress Reduction

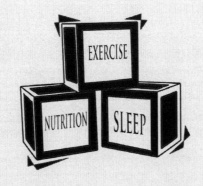

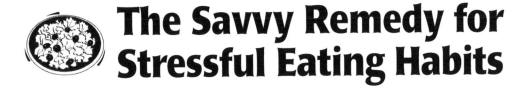 The Savvy Remedy for Stressful Eating Habits

---

In This Chapter

➤ Taking stock in stress eating

➤ Breaking stress eating habits

➤ Healthier eating for stress resistance

➤ Benefits of an if-then plan

In this chapter, you'll have a chance to examine some of the eating habits people have when under pressure. You'll identify the triggers that get you eating because of stress. Plus, you'll learn ways to break old patterns and build new ones that reduce your stress level, make you more stress resistant, and help you cope with major stressors in the long run.

Stressed to the Max, Filled to the Gills

Most mornings Marla hits the ground running, grabs a doughnut, and scurries out the door, coffee sloshing on her dress as her car whines its way to work. Midday, she eats a taco at her computer or skips lunch altogether, digging through piles of work on her desk. Evenings, she rushes home and throws a frozen dinner in the oven for her two children, who need help with their homework before bedtime. The next morning, she hops on the (not so merry) merry-go-round and repeats the same routine until week's end.

Stress has a powerful effect on appetite. But does eating reduce stress? Fat chance. What you eat can help you cope better or make your stress worse. Under strain, some people eat more, others less. Both patterns can be problematic. Studies show that chronic stress leads to poor nutritional choices and causes fluctuations in the amount of food you eat.

Trending Now from the Smart Files

Here are some statistics on the eating habits of the American public:

The US Department of Agriculture (USDA) reports that Americans eat 40 percent of their meals outside the home; 50 percent of Americans skip breakfast, 25 percent skip lunch, and 60 percent get one-fifth of their calories from snacking.

➤ In 2011, the National Center for Health Statistics reported that over one-third of grown-ups in the United States are overweight, and 34 percent are obese.

➤ Asked by scientists to give their main barriers to healthier eating habits, 28 percent of adults say they don't have enough time, 20 percent say healthy foods are too expensive, and 20 percent prefers to indulge themselves.

Stress Vocab

Stress Eating, also called emotional eating, is the practice of consuming a large amount of junk food activated not by hunger, but by an attempt to comfort stressful emotions such as worry, anger, boredom, frustration, loneliness, fear, anxiety, or depression.

Stress and Your Appetite

Do you eat when you're not hungry? Do you avoid stressful situations by eating? Do you use food as a reward? Or do you grab, gulp, and go without paying attention to your hunger or taste? If you're a stress eater, reaching for comfort foods is such an automatic habit you don't realize you're doing it. And when you're slammed, you're more likely to eat fattening, high-calorie foods and to feel like your eating is out of control. Fast foods, frozen dinners, and comfort foods are convenient and appealing.

When you're stressed, eating becomes a task to complete instead of an experience to enjoy. You're more likely to eat quickly and to overeat without really tasting your food. If you gulp down a Diet Coke, hamburger, and fries so you can hurry back to the office, you're stress eating, a type of eating that raises your stress level. After all, what would life be like without Starbucks, Burger King, and Ben & Jerry's?

Are You the Five-Napkin Burger Type?

Rick is tense and wary, alert to every sound and sudden movement. His bills are stacking up and he's falling further behind in a hospital administrator job that he hates. As he walks through the main entrance at work, his heart is pounding; his hands and jaw are clenched. The first thing he does is amble to the break room and reach for a pastry.

Are you a junk food junkie? If so, you could be feeding your stress instead of managing it. No wonder you might seek out comfort foods when you're stressed out. Stress and certain foods go hand in hand: sweets, starches like mashed potatoes, fats, and salty foods like French fries. These foods act like a natural tranquilizer that calms you down in times of peril. Research shows that glucose—natural body sugars that are released from your liver and muscles—must be replenished after a stressor has passed. So the more glucose you release in reacting to stress, the hungrier you'll be *after* the stressor. Cheeseburger, anyone?

The Stress-Eating Cycle

It's not natural for your body to be stressed on an ongoing basis. And it's not healthy to use food for comfort. Still, experts estimate that 75 percent of overeating is caused by stress-related emotional states. In the long run, eating for comfort traps you in a hard-to-break eating cycle that adds to your stress level and can result in serious health problems such as heart disease, high blood pressure, diabetes, and obesity, as well as emotional problems such as depression and anxiety. In other words, what feels like a satisfying solution in the moment becomes a bigger problem later on.

Under stress, your body uses up essential vitamins and minerals. Bad eating habits dampen your body's ability to fend off stress. To offset this pattern, it's important to prepare your body ahead of time with good food. When you're equipped with nutritional armor, your body reacts to stressful events and then returns to normal.

Stress Eating and Your Cortisol Cocktail

When your nutrition is in the gutter, chronically elevated levels of cortisol keep your internal alarm system on around the clock. You'll remember from Chapter 1 that high doses of cortisol prompt your body to overreact to normal daily stress, causing your blood pressure and pulse rate to climb. To fight off stress, cortisol uses up antioxidants such as vitamins A, B, C, and E, and depletes your body of essential minerals such as calcium, iron, zinc, and magnesium—the very fuel it needs to fight off stress. A large amount of cortisol also makes you crave foods high in fat, sugar, and salt—a craving that results in stress eating, a secondary problem that causes further damage to your body.

What Are Your Stress-Eating Triggers?

Chronic stress distracts you from monitoring your eating habits. Start asking yourself how you eat when your stress meter tops the charts. Do you munch on chocolate? Binge on junk food like potato chips and French fries? Or impose strict eating rules and deprive yourself of food?

Shock Absorber

Think back over your day or week and notice the difference between stress hunger and true physical hunger. From now on, pay closer attention to what triggers you to eat, and identify patterns of emotional eating. How do you feel when you stress eat? Sad maybe? Or bored, lonely, or scared? Use your stress journal to record any association you have at the time you're eating to stress, negative thoughts, or worries. You might find that you stress eat the night before a big presentation, when worried about a family member's health or about a problem at work. Once you realize you're stress eating, develop a preset plan that will curb this tendency and help you deal more directly with the stressor. (See the section at the end of this chapter on how to create a preset plan.) Being more mindful of your hunger will help you regulate when, what, and how much you eat and keep it in line with your body's needs.

Restocking Your Body with Stress-Busting Foods

When you're burning the candle at both ends, a well-nourished body has a stronger stress-resistance shield. Once you adopt healthy eating habits, it will become second nature, and you'll automatically reach for the apple instead of the Danish. To help your body fend off stress, certain foods can fortify you, while others deplete your body's resistance. The next section presents some foods to stay away from and some to include in your stress-busting diet.

Avoid Caffeine

Cut down on caffeinated drinks that tax your nervous system, interfere with sleep, and dehydrate you. Replace Red Bulls, Diet Cokes, and Dunkin' Donuts coffee with bottled water, protein smoothies, fruit juices, or herbal teas. For instance, in contrast to coffee, which boosts your cortisol level, did you know that black or green tea lowers it? That's right. These teas increase levels of relaxing chemicals in the brain.

Eat Complex Carbs

Introduce complex carbs into your diet. A bowl of warm oatmeal can boost your serotonin level as can other complex carbs. Slowly digested high-fiber foods like whole grain breads, cereals, and pastas will stabilize blood sugar levels.

Stress Vocab

Serotonin is a calming brain chemical—activated by certain foods—that boosts mood and creates a sense of well-being.

Watch Your Sugar Intake

Shun simple carbs like quickly digested refined sugars that give you a fast serotonin high (and a quick crash). Too much sugar can cause rapid fluctuations in blood sugar levels and poor concentration, triggering stress. I hate to say it, but Mom knew best when she said, "Eat your veggies." Try eating more fruits and vegetables, which are digested more slowly and give you energy over the long haul.

Introduce Omega-3 Foods

Substitute high-fat meats with omega-3 fatty acids found in fish such as salmon and tuna. Omega-3 fatty acids protect against heart disease and prevent surges in stress hormones. Studies show that foods containing omega-3 fatty acids even help relieve mild depression. In addition to seafood, nuts, seeds, and oils such as canola, flax, and soybean provide these benefits.

Restore Vitamins and Minerals

Replenish your body with the vitamins and minerals that it loses during bouts of stress. Eating well-balanced meals high in antioxidants and nutritional supplements of vitamins A, B, C, and E resupplies your body with the nutrients it needs.

Almonds restore vitamins B and E. The B vitamins strengthen your nervous system and help with stress-related fatigue by alleviating foggy thoughts. You can get those benefits from asparagus, spinach, and potatoes as well. Vitamin C sources like oranges and foods that contain

Truth Serum

Research links B vitamins to preserving memory, and enhancing mood and cognitive mastery. Studies also show that adults who take high doses of B complex supplements for one month are less subject to stress and perform higher on mental tests than those not taking supplements.

magnesium—such as spinach or soybeans—reduce cortisol hormone levels and strengthen your immune system.

Use Low-Fat Dairy Products

Fill your fridge with low-fat dairy products and yogurt to restore lost calcium and magnesium that your body uses up to fend off stress, help you relax, and avoid mood swings. Stay away from saturated fats and trans-fats. Eat meats, poultry, and fish that are baked, broiled, or grilled.

Eat Healthy Snacks

Many snacks such as cheese puffs or potato chips are loaded with salty ingredients and artificial additives. These empty nutrients don't give you the fuel you need to offset stress. Your body doesn't recognize these artificial ingredients as natural and reacts defensively, putting undue strain on your immune system. Stock your car and office desk with high-protein, low-calorie snacks to prevent blood sugar dips and stress-related fatigue. Nibble on protein bars or trail mix. I keep granola bars in my office desk drawer just in case. Your body needs protein when you're stressed because it uses up more amino acids to produce the additional stress hormones.

Buy Healthy Munchies

Munch on raw fruits, nuts, and vegetables. Apple wedges, celery, carrot sticks, or sunflower seeds contain stress-reducing compounds called flavonoids. And pistachios counteract the impact of stress and keep blood pressure down.

Stress Vocab

Flavonoids, sometimes called vitamin P, are antioxidants found in certain plants such as tomatoes, cabbage, pears, blueberries, and apricots. They're believed to strengthen blood vessels, prevent cancers and heart disease, protect cells from oxygen damage, and reduce excessive inflammation throughout the body.

Manage Your Stress with Good Nutrition

There are some simple steps you can follow to help you use good nutrition and manage your bouts with stress.

Start Slow

Refrain from abruptly turning your dietary habits upside down. Introducing healthier foods slowly will increase your chances of success. Take it one meal at a time, replacing unhealthy foods with more nutritional choices such as serving baked chicken instead of fried chicken. Set limits on when you eat, only at three set mealtimes a day for example, and stick to them. Gauge your appetite by the clock, not by your emotions.

Avoid Strict Restraint

If you think of healthy eating as dieting or depriving yourself of the foods you love, it backfires. And studies back that up. Research shows that trying to control your weight by following fad diets, skipping meals, rigidly avoiding certain foods, or ignoring hunger pangs eventually causes you to eat everything in sight. Eat sensibly. Healthy eating doesn't require torture or deprivation. If you like ice cream or yogurt, choose a low-fat version. Moderation in food portions and frequency of eating plus well-balanced meals are the key. So eat healthier, smaller portions, and eat slower.

Stop Skipping Meals

Avoid jogging out the door in the morning, jostling a cup of java like Marla does. If you're in a hurry, try making a protein shake. That's what I have for breakfast every morning, harried or with time to kill. You can purchase powdered protein at any health food store. Throw it in the blender with a frozen banana and skim milk. And voila! You can even carry it with you. The earlier in the day you stock your body with nutritional foods, the more armored you are against stress as it comes. Skipping breakfast makes it harder for your body to maintain stable blood sugar levels throughout the busy morning. To avoid skipping lunch, carry a healthy meal from home and eat lunch outside with a friend under a shade tree or in a quiet park.

Portion Meals

Avoid drinking from milk cartons, eating out of ice cream containers, or snacking from potato chip bags. When you cannot measure your food, you automatically eat more, which contributes to unwanted weight gain and obesity. Snacks and meals should be portioned on a plate or in a bowl. Then, put the cartons, containers, and bags away. Studies show that when you use smaller plates, you eat less.

Practice Mindful Eating

Steer clear of grabbing, gulping, and going—eating while standing, driving, on the run, or watching TV. Treat mealtime as a singular activity with value in its own right. Sitting down, eating slowly, and chewing a few times before swallowing, appreciating textures, aromas, and flavors of your food helps you relax and enjoy your meal as well as aid in digestion. Plus, it gives your stomach time to tell your brain when it's full, and you will be less likely to eat as much.

Recharging Your Batteries

Taste your food in a completely different way with a mindful eating exercise (See Chapter 12 for more mindfulness exercises).

During your next meal, sit down and give the food your full attention. Think about where the food was grown and how it sprouted from a seed to a vegetable. Pause before starting to eat, noticing the colors and textures while inhaling the aroma. Chew slowly and deliberately, being mindful of each bite. Chew two or three more times than you usually do to taste it fully, savoring the texture and temperature of each morsel. For example, instead of tasting tuna salad, discover the flavor, texture, and coolness of celery as it crushes against your teeth, the bursting tartness of pickles, and the blending of the tuna and green lettuce. Take a sip of a beverage and be aware of the sensation against your tongue and as it slides down the back of your throat. Linger for awhile after your meal, giving your stomach time to digest the food and to tell your brain you've finished.

Inventory Your Kitchen

Scientists say that surrounding yourself with healthy foods goes a long way to getting them into your stomach. When you're under the gun, your appetite has a mind of its own and focuses on what's in front of you. So purge your fridge and cabinets of unhealthy foods that tempt you. If you don't have high-fat sugars like ice cream in the freezer or salty chips in the cupboard, you're more likely to reach for healthier fare. So make sure you stock your kitchen with healthy munchies and nutritional foods that you purchase and prepare yourself instead of buying foods that are bad for you or fast foods that you bring home. Plan a special time to clean out your kitchen cabinets and fridge and get rid of all the junk food.

Change Your Routines

Remove yourself from settings that you associate with binge eating. After a stressful day, instead of plopping in front of your TV with a case of beer or carton of ice cream, plan something different. Get in the habit of rewarding yourself after a long day with a healthier activity: walk your dog, play computer games with the kids, check your e-mail, go to the gym, visit a friend, listen to relaxing music, get a massage, or write in your stress journal.

Breaking Bad Stress Habits

Ever have a small setback or fall into a bad mood and throw your resolutions to the wind? Ever say to hell with it because you blew your eating plan when you polished off that chocolate bar in the morning, so you figure you might as well have dessert after dinner?

Sometimes when you're grappling with eating habits, relapse is part of the package. But when you have a setback, it's tempting to condemn yourself and chuck the whole idea. This impulsive reaction is an attempt to bring quick relief to your misery of failing. So you seek comfort in the very thing you're trying to conquer. Truth be told, this attitude, called the what-the-hell effect, adds heartache on top of heartache.

The What-the-Hell Effect When You Slip

Studies show that especially among people trying to break a habit, disappointment triggers a what-the-hell attitude and turns a minor slip into a major relapse. It lets you return to the bad habit, which comforted you in the first place.

Truth Serum

Dr. Janet Polivy at the University of Toronto put the what-the-hell attitude under scientific scrutiny. She served dieters unusually large slices of pizza to compare with non-dieters who were served smaller slices. Then, when a plateful of cookies came their way, dieters were inclined to eat more of the sweets than non-dieters. Turns out the dieters saw the excessive pizza that they'd already eaten as a license to pig out.

After being provoked into a bad mood, you're more likely to give up your goals and engage in risky behavior so you don't have to keep feeling bad about failing. The bad mood eclipses your goal of breaking a bad habit. And the what-the-hell attitude gives you a way out—permission to backslide with whatever behavior you're trying to change. Studies show that two preventive strategies can keep you from falling into the what-the-hell pit:

> ➤ Treat yourself with compassion after your shortcomings get the better of you

> ➤ Have an if-then plan

Recharging Your Batteries

You don't have to berate yourself to make successful changes. Studies show when people have setbacks—whether they're trying to taper off stress eating or stay on an exercise plan—accepting exactly where they are without criticizing themselves makes them more likely to succeed.

Plus, if you think of foregoing that cigarette or extra piece of cake as self-care instead of self-denial, it'll keep you from adding insult to injury. See your shortcomings for what they are: habits, behavior patterns, or just plain mistakes. When you accept your shortcomings, you cut your stress in half. Then you deal with the painful experience, not the added bad feelings from judging yourself.

From Mission Impossible to Mission Accomplished

How many times have you resolved to eat healthier and exercise more? Then two months down the road, your vows have become a distant memory. Well, you're not alone. There was a time when I ate anything and everything I wanted, smoked like a chimney, and shunned exercise. I wasn't exactly on the road to health, happiness, and longevity. Oh sure, I promised over and over again to stop smoking, eat better, and start exercising. But my endless excuses always trumped the empty promises. Until I found a magic solution that helped me stick to my goals. It's called the if-then plan—a surefire strategy to resist temptation and build healthy habits by sticking to the action part of a challenging goal.

The built-in strategy of the if-then plan inoculates you from the self-defeating what-the-hell attitude. New York University researcher Peter Gollwitzer found that having an action plan for what you intend to do before you encounter a situation triples the chances of accomplishing your goals. In one study, he found that 91 percent of people who used his if-then plan stuck to their exercise plan compared to 39 percent of those who didn't use the formula. You've got to admit those are pretty impressive odds.

And the if-then plan has worked magic in my life. My plan for exercise went from a vague, "I will exercise more," to applying the "If *x* happens, then I'll do *y*." The *x* is the situation, and *y* is the action you'll take when *x* occurs. Plugging my idle vow to exercise into the formula looked like this: "Every Tuesday and Thursday mornings at 8:00 a.m., I'll meet my personal trainer at the gym for a one-hour workout." Translating my abstract goal into a specific action plan helped me get moving, and I've been at it for many years now.

The if-then plan is not really magic. Of course, you knew that all along. So why does it work? Experts say it takes about one month to break an old habit and replace it with a good one. But being specific about when and where you will act on your goal (the "if"), automatically alerts your brain to be on the lookout for a specific situation (the "if") and the action that must follow (the "then"). Without an automatic reminder, your brain gets sidetracked from remembering the intended behavior and constantly calculates whether an event is the right one to carry out the intended action.

Let's say you're trying to avoid fried foods. So you make an if-then plan that might look something like this: "If I see fried foods on a restaurant menu, then I'll avoid them." Now you have hardwired the situation, being at a restaurant and seeing fried foods, directly to the action, avoid them. Your brain develops a heightened vigilance for the "if" situation. Once triggered, it is automatically equipped with the prepared response of avoiding fried foods (the "then" action). Armed with an if-then plan, you are more apt to carry out your goal without struggling to consciously think about it. Now you will be able to kiss willpower good-bye and proclaim, "Mission accomplished!"

The Doctor Of Calm Is In

You can't hit a target you cannot see, and you cannot see a target you do not have.

—Zig Zigler

In the space below, set a target goal to change a stress-eating habit. Then triple your chances of follow-through by plugging the goal into the if-then formula:

Target: If X Happens (the event), Then I'll do Y (My Action)

My prescription: Instead of diet pills or yo-yo diets, take a dose of the if-then plan. Break one bad eating habit a month for the next six months. Continue with your plan until cravings subside. Here's to outsmarting your stress!

CHAPTER 7

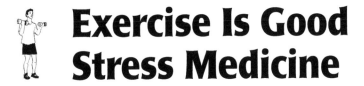

Exercise Is Good Stress Medicine

In This Chapter

➤ The benefits of exercise

➤ Evaluating your exercise regimen

➤ The importance of stretching

➤ Choosing the best workout for you

In this chapter, you'll learn the antistress benefits of exercise. You'll have a chance to examine your exercise habits and find the right regimen for you. Even if there are physical capabilities that limit you, you'll discover ways of moving to reduce stress and improve your daily functioning.

Exercise for the Health of It

You've heard it said a million times before. By now you're probably sick of hearing it, so I apologize before hitting you with this. But the fact is that vigorous physical exercise is a powerful tool against stress. The other sad truth is that as many as 40 percent of Americans prefer lying on their duff to exercising. But don't think like comedian Joan Rivers who teased, "I don't exercise. If God had wanted me to bend over, He would have put diamonds on the floor."

"Yeah, yeah," you might say, "I'll get around to it when I have the time." Most of us know that exercise is essential for our physical and mental health, but we don't really *know* it. Unfortunately, it sometimes takes a crisis before it sinks in and we're willing to do anything about it.

So before blowing off this subject, please indulge me as I dig a little deeper into the facts. Then after you've let me sound off, you can decide whether to plop back into your La-Z-Boy or put on your running shoes.

Are You a Couch Potato?

Okay, I'll admit it. Working out sucks. There, I said it. But let's look at the alternative. Long stretches of sitting without enough exercise endanger your heart and the cells of your body. Most people gain weight because of stress, not by overeating. Studies show that being a couch potato is as bad or worse than smoking and actually cuts your life expectancy. According to a 2011 American Cancer Society study, women who sat more than six hours per day were 34 percent more likely to die than those who were more active. The same figure for men was 18 percent.

Truth Serum

Wise up! Mounting evidence shows conclusively that one of the biggest health stressors is sitting too much. Experts say that parking yourself for more than four to six hours a day puts you at an 80 percent greater risk of dying from cardiovascular disease. Most Americans spend an average of ten hours a day in a car, at a computer, or in front of TV. If you sit a lot, you're more likely to build stress, gain weight, and develop heart disease and diabetes. A little exercise goes a long way to fuel your brain's stress buffers and prevent heart disease.

On the flip side, scientists tell us that regular exercise builds resistance to stress. Danish researchers found that people who exercise at any intensity for just seventeen minutes a day feel 61 percent less stressed. That's because exercise increases blood flow and oxygen throughout the body, lowers blood pressure, and improves overall mental and physical health.

Study after study shows that exercise strengthens the heart, brain, muscles, bones, immune system, and psychological immunity to life's stressors. Plus, a good workout makes you feel good. After just twenty minutes of vigorous exercise, your brain releases endocannabinoids that give you a feeling of well-being, sometimes called a natural high, and gives you a positive outlook on life.

Consistent exercise has a host of other antistress benefits including the following:

➤ It gives you a positive outlet for frustration, anger, and irritability.

➤ It reduces your skeletal muscle tension and helps you relax.

➤ It decreases depression and anxiety.

➤ It elevates your mood and raises your energy level.

➤ It sharpens your mental alertness and concentration.

➤ It strengthens your immune system.

➤ It regulates your weight gain and muscle tone.

➤ It boosts your self-worth and confidence.

➤ It deepens your restful sleep.

Stress Vocab

Endocannabinoids are morphine-like neurotransmitters secreted by the brain during exercise and function as the body's natural painkillers, creating a sense of euphoria.

Trending Now from the Smart Files

Here are some statistics showing that exercise inoculates against stress-related illnesses:

➤ The American College of Sports Medicine reports that workers who exercise a minimum of 45 minutes a week take 25 to 50 percent fewer sick days.

➤ Duke University researchers say that exercise and stress management training reduces a heart patient's emotional distress, depression, and cardiovascular risk more than routine medical care does.

➤ British scientists in the journal *Lancet Neurology* report that middle-agers who exercise at least twice a week are 60 percent less likely to develop Alzheimer's disease than couch potatoes.

➤ A University of Illinois study shows that simple aerobic exercise—such as walking forty-five minutes a day, three times a week—improves memory and executive-control functions in your brain by 20 percent.

➤ The American College of Sports Medicine reports that twenty minutes of moderate exercise creates a rise in mood-enhancing neurotransmitters and a feel-good afterglow that can last up to twelve hours.

Get Out of Your La-Z-Boy and Live Ten Years Longer

If you're like most people, when life's hassles land you down in the dumps, you want instant relief. The first thing you reach for to feel better is a beer, cigarette, or piece of chocolate. Then you wiggle your body deeper into the sofa. The last thing you want to do is exercise.

But when you read the stats on stress and exercise, why wouldn't you want to work up a sweat two or three times a week? We know for a fact that active people have less depression and anxiety than sedentary people. But if you're still not convinced to start pumping iron, what if I said exercise could add ten years to your life? Would that make you put on your sweats? Well, that's exactly what new research shows.

Truth Serum

Researchers at the University of Illinois just might have found the fountain of youth. They report that fitness training changes your molecular and cellular building blocks. A year of exercise, they say, gives a seventy-year-old the brain connectivity of a thirty-year-old, improving memory and the ability to plan, deal with ambiguity, and multitask. Scientists also find that adults ages fifty to eighty who spend a year doing aerobic exercise regularly increase the size of their brain in the area of the hippocampus—the area responsible for short-term memory and spatial navigation.

In her book *Stress Less: The New Science That Shows Women How to Rejuvenate the Body and the Mind*, Thea Singer summarizes the extensive research on exercise and stress from a cellular level. She shows without doubt that chronic stress increases the rate at which your cells age by ten years and that exercise holds the key to long, healthy living.

Moderately brisk workouts reverse the aging process by slowing the aging of your cells, combating life's stressors, and extending your life. Here's how: Physical activity of any kind detoxifies your body by metabolizing brain chemicals that your body produces during stressful times. Exercise neutralizes adrenaline, thyroxin, cortisol, and other hormones that accumulate in your bloodstream when the fight-or-flight response gets activated.

Latest research questions the popular notion that a rush of endorphins creates the high you get from exercising. But while the neurotransmitter role is still unclear, one thing is for sure: physical activity fuels your brain's stress buffers, strengthening your ability to respond to stress.

The more sedentary you are, the less your body will be prepared to resist stress when it comes. By contrast, regular exercise forces your body's physical systems to work together, giving it practice to fend off stress, build immunity to future stressors, and make you more stress resistant. In other words, the more exercise you get, the less affected you will be by stress in the future and the slower your cells will age.

Changing Your Tune about Exercise

As you can see, exercise is the ticket for less stress, better health, and longer life. The movement involved in any physical activity evaporates daily tensions that have built in your mind and body. When you add up all the pluses of exercising, it can change your tune.

The specific form of exercise doesn't matter all that much as long as you're consistent and stick to it. High-energy activities such as weight lifting, racquetball, aerobics, laps in a pool, running, or dancing are beneficial. And so are low-energy activities such as walking, gardening, bicycling, yoga, tai chi, or stretching. So get moving. Stand, walk, run, dance, stretch, or bend. Just moving around can make a difference in your stress health. But make sure you challenge yourself within the range of your physical capabilities.

Recharging Your Batteries

A little exercise goes a long way. Scientists say that just fifteen minutes of exercise a day can help with stress and prevent heart disease. But they recommend at least one-half hour three times a week of cardio exercise. Even if you can't do a rigorous workout, just moving around can cut your risk of sudden cardiac arrest by 92 percent. Experts say just being on your feet at your desk instead of sitting can help. Simply not sitting gives you the benefits of exercise, plus, sweating reduces your stress level.

Stretching: Your Stress Offensive

Trish, my kick-butt personal trainer, is always telling me how important it is to stretch. She reminds me that stretching before and after a rigorous workout prevents injury and relieves pain associated with an injury. Even if you don't exercise regularly, Trish recommends stretching as a stress reliever at least three times a week.

I want to share with you some of the stretches that Trish makes me do (uh, I mean asks me to do) before exercising two or three times a week when I meet with her. Trish separates the simplest and safest types of stretching into two categories: dynamic stretches and static stretches.

Stress Vocab

Dynamic stretches are slow, controlled movements of joints through a full range of motion such as raising your arms over your head and lowering them back down.

Static stretches are stretches that focus on specific muscles such as the shoulders while the rest of the body is at rest.

Trish cites research on strength and conditioning that shows dynamic stretches are the best for warming up as a lead-in to static stretches, which are best for cooling down. As you begin stretching, remember to pay attention to your body. If a motion is painful or if you have a chronic condition or injury, alter your stretches so that you are not pushing or overexerting yourself.

Dynamic Stretches

According to Trish, you can increase a joint's or muscle's range of motion by holding the stretch for at least thirty seconds during dynamic stretching. Begin a stretch and once you feel the pull, stay there and breathe deeply. You may feel the pull release some, and at that point you can exhale and move further into the stretch. If you are not accustomed to stretching, try to relax all other parts of your body while your attention is set on a tight area. For example, while you're holding a hamstring stretch, stay relaxed in your shoulders, neck, and face.

Start by raising your arms over your head and lowering them back down. As you raise your arms, focus on increasing the height of your arms at varying angles: to the front, side, back, or anywhere in between.

For the legs and hips, start by marching in place or walking. Once the feeling of warmth in the muscles sets in and the joints feel loose, take longer strides and pick up your knees a bit higher. Think about extending your knees straight (but not locked) with each stride, and extend your legs from your hip behind, pushing off from your back leg as if you're skating on ice.

Dynamic stretching for eight to ten minutes can be a sufficient amount of time to warm up your muscles and joints to get more benefit from static stretches.

Static Stretches

As you move into static stretching, Trish cautions that these stretches should never hurt or cause you pain. So make sure that you practice them slowly and gently.

The muscles in your lower back have multiple layers and are attached to your hips, spine, and ribs. Pain in this region is usually a result of tight hamstrings. These muscles may have been overused or improperly used while lifting packages or moving objects. Bending over to clean or garden also can induce sore muscles of your lower back. As long as you don't have a lower-back injury, the following exercise can help relieve tightness there:

Back flat on the floor and abdominal muscles tightened, bring both of your legs to your chest. Hug your arms around the back of your thighs and bend your knees. Keep your shoulders and neck relaxed. Breathe deeply. After exhaling, raise your head and shoulders to curl up like a ball, again staying contracted in your abdomen. Breathe deeply and remain curled up like a ball for thirty seconds. Return to lying on your back with your legs stretched out.

Contract your abdominal muscles and lift one leg up to your chest. Wrap both hands behind your thigh and hold this position, breathing deeply. During this static stretch, concentrate on lengthening the leg that is still extended on the floor. Tighten your buttocks on that side and notice a stretch at the front of your hip. Keep your abdominals engaged to increase lengthening across your lower back. After holding this position for thirty seconds, bend your leg and lower your knee across your body to the opposite side. Do this carefully, slowly, and only as far as you feel it is beneficial. It would be ideal if you could reach your bent knee to the floor, but go only as far as you can without overexerting yourself.

Shock Absorber

Pilates is a gentle way to begin an exercise regimen. When stress deals you a blow, your body automatically tightens, hunches, or recoils in ways you might not be aware of. Pilates is your best defense to restore your body to its original fitness whether you're a new mom, retiree, or jock. Pilates makes you more aware of how you sit, stand, lift, and move during daily activities. And it helps you maintain proper posture when you're driving, walking, typing at your computer, brushing your teeth, cooking, or climbing stairs. Pilates exercises improve range of motion, flexibility, circulation, and abdominal strength. They decrease back, neck, and joint pain due to stress. Plus, they make better posture a daily habit. The best way to understand proper Pilates positioning is to take a class. Classes are held in every major city across the United States in gyms, community centers, and community colleges.

In this stretch, turn your head in the opposite direction of your bent knee and try to keep both shoulder blades on the floor. As always, hold this stretch and try to progress it for at least thirty seconds. Return to your back and repeat the stretch on the other side.

Stress Vocab

Pilates (pronounced puh-LAH-teez) is a system of strengthening and stretching exercises designed by Joseph Pilates in the 1960s to develop the body's core, mobilize the spine, build flexibility, lengthen muscles, and raise body awareness.

A Taste of Pilates

Here's a taste of Pilates positioning that Trish instructs me to do from time to time:

On a mat, take the position lying on your back and bring your attention to your shoulder blades. Try to spread them out wide on your mat as if you're trying to flatten them to the floor. Easy now, you want a gentle stretch, not jerking or pulling. This position should make it feel like you're opening across your collarbone. You might feel stretching in the muscles of your front shoulders and chest.

Gently slide your shoulder blades down toward your hips, away from your ears. Make sure you keep hip bones level. Now try to lengthen the back of your neck as if there's a string attached to the top of your head and someone is gently pulling on it. Lengthen your spine at the back of your neck, down between your shoulder blades, through the lower back all the way to your tailbone. You might feel like you've already grown a couple inches!

While holding this position, try raising your arms slowly overhead. Your shoulder blades may automatically lift toward your ears. Don't let them! Stay strong in the muscles around them in order to keep them spread out on the floor. Lower your arms to your sides with the same awareness. Repeat the arm pattern five to ten times slowly while breathing deeply.

Choosing the Best Exercise for You

The activities you choose should match your physical capabilities, and it is important to consult with your physician before embarking on an exercise program. Once you've done that, there are a number of points for you to consider when choosing the right exercise for you.

Start Small

Choose an easily accessible activity that requires minor preparation like brisk walking. While a twenty- to thirty-minute workout might get you that feel-good rush, take baby steps to get there. Start with five minutes of walking or stretching and gradually increase the amount of time as you build your endurance.

Take It Slow

Don't go from low-energy activities like watching TV to high-energy activities like kickboxing in the blink of an eye. Moving too fast can lead to injury and defeat. When you take it one step at a time and build your fitness gradually, you're more likely to stick with it. Start by taking the stairs instead of the elevator or parking a distance from the mall and walking.

Choose Something You Enjoy

The best exercise program is the one you enjoy doing. It's next to impossible to sustain an exercise program that you don't like. Thinking of exercise as another item on your to-do list creates rather than relieves stress.

Make your exercise a fun activity that you look forward to instead of one that you dread. Choosing something you enjoy will make it easier to get going. If you hate doing push-ups but love gardening, start with weeding, digging in the dirt, or planting a favorite flower.

Recharging Your Batteries

Exercise in an environment different from the one you're in all day. If you work around people, a large exercise class might not be your cup of tea. If you work alone, the social interaction of team sports or an aerobics class might be just what the doctor ordered. After a stressful day, you might find exercising in a stress-free environment—like jogging in a quiet park or taking a nature hike in the woods—more appealing than running along a hectic city street.

Find an Exercise Buddy

Companionship during exercise is a powerful incentive to stay motivated. Joining a walking group or working out with a friend, family member, or coworker will give you encouragement to get you going and will push you harder to stick with it. Contact with others during exercise gives you the added benefit of social interaction and can make the activity more enjoyable.

Think Beyond Your Limitations

If you have physical limitations, don't let them stall your exercise program. If you have a bad back, low-impact activities are your best bet. Even if you're wheelchair bound or bedridden, you can do modified exercises such as arm or leg lifts. Experts recommend that people with painful conditions like fibromyalgia or arthritis try low-energy exercise such as swimming and tai chi for pain relief.

Try Not to Go Overboard

Studies show that moderate exercise is more beneficial than overexercise. People who get carried away and overdo it wash out the health and longevity advantages of working out. The body cells of compulsive, heavy-duty exercisers age just as fast and their immune systems function just as poorly as those who never get off the couch.

Don't Park It for Too Long

When you schedule time for regular exercise like you would for a meeting, you're more likely to keep at it. And the excuse, "I don't have time" won't hold water. If you hear yourself say, "What the hell, I've already missed two days of exercise; I might as well skip the whole week," avoid going back to the habit you're trying to break: lethargy. Remind yourself you've fallen into the what-the-hell pit and consult Chapter 6 about an if-then plan to dig your way out.

"Rx from Dr. Bryan"

The Doctor Of Calm Is In

Those who think they have not time for bodily exercise will sooner or later have to find time for illness.

—Edward Stanley

Now that you have the scoop on stress and exercise, which is it: plopping in the La-Z-Boy or hopping on the treadmill? For your health's sake, I hope it's the latter. If you've been looking for the fountain of youth, you won't find it in a chill pill or through cosmetic surgery. It's contained in your StairMaster, your swim suit, or your dancing shoes. All you have to do to turn back the clock and stay fit is get busy. My prescription: Make the effort to develop the new habit of making exercise the first medicine you reach for—like going to the gym instead of to happy hour—when you're feeling stressed. And you'll start to feel like that's just what the doctor ordered. Here's to outsmarting your stress!

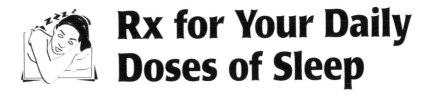

CHAPTER 8

Rx for Your Daily Doses of Sleep

In This Chapter

➤ Restorative benefits of sleep

➤ Evaluating your sleep regimen

➤ Improving your sleep habits

➤ Power napping

In this chapter, you'll discover the benefits of sleep. You'll have a chance to reexamine some of your sleep habits, learn ways to break old patterns, and build new ones that will make you more stress resistant. You might even consider power napping or at the very least getting more shut-eye at night.

The Trifecta of Stress Reduction

I don't know anyone who doesn't want less stress in their lives. But it doesn't magically happen, and it doesn't happen overnight. It's easy to lose sight of the fact that if you want to reduce your stress, you have to change your lifestyle. Although it takes time and patience, a healthy lifestyle makes you more invincible to major life stressors.

Scientists insist they have discovered the winning combination for a long, calm, happy life—the holy grail of stress reduction. This trio of lifestyle habits gives you the stamina to withstand just about any curveball life throws at you. I call them the trifecta of stress reduction:

➤ Healthy eating habits

➤ Regular exercise

➤ Adequate sleep

You won't be the bionic man or woman; you won't be a Pee-Wee Herman, either. But making changes in these three areas can build the armor you need to cope with everyday problems, reduce your stress, and improve your outlook on life. You've already read about the importance of healthy eating and regular exercise. Now let's turn to the third member of the antistress trinity—adequate sleep.

Are You Getting Enough Snooze Time?

Many of us take sleep for granted, yet sleep's restorative nature makes it one of the best stress remedies. It has been said that the best bridge between despair and hope is a good night's sleep. And it's true. A good night's sleep can give you a whole new lease on life. Experts say the average person needs seven to eight hours of sleep a night for optimal health. Those who doze eight or more hours are less stressed out, have fewer colds and viruses, and live longer.

Sleepless in Seattle

It's not just Seattle that's missing out on sleep. Surveys report that half of Americans say stress interferes with sleep. The National Sleep Foundation reports that the average American sleeps less than seven hours a night because of stress. What about you? Are you getting enough snooze time? If you're overly stressed, chances are you're not.

Truth Serum

About 3 percent of the population makes up what scientists call short sleepers. They are a rare group who sleep only three hours a night and then hit the gym. They are resourceful and successful, and they thrive on little sleep. But for most of us, getting either too much or not enough sleep can spell trouble. A long-term sleep study shows that people who sleep less than six or more than eight hours at night have a decline in brain function equivalent to aging four to seven years.

Sleep is restorative. When you don't doze enough, sleep deprivation lowers your resistance to stress and harms your brain. Research shows that being sleep deprived interferes with memory and learning. Your brain moves slower. You're more forgetful. Your attention is short-circuited, and you're grumpier. Plus, you're more likely to nod off at your desk. Studies also show that those who don't get enough sleep are at increased risk of heart attack or stroke, and their risk of death from heart disease more than doubles. Lack of sleep is linked to depression, impaired immune system function, weight gain, hypertension, and type 2 diabetes.

Trending Now from the Smart Files

Here is a wake-up call on sleep stats:

➤ 52 percent of Americans report that stress interferes with sleep

➤ 36 percent of the US population has sleep stress more than once a week

➤ 45 percent of Americans toss and turn because of their mate's sleep stress

➤ 50 to 70 million Americans have chronic sleep disorders

The Sleep-Stress Tug-of-War

Stress never rests and it doesn't keep office hours. It's with you wherever you go 24/7, which creates a tug-of-war between sleep and stress. When you're stressed, it elevates your stress hormones, disrupting your sleep cycle which makes it harder to sleep. When you can't sleep, it increases your stress level.

The timing of many of your life activities has a lot to do with how much shut-eye you get. Exercise midday aids your sleep, but exercise right before bedtime can actually disrupt it. Chugging a Red Bull to pick you up in late afternoon could cause you to toss and turn when you fall into bed. When you take your naps, do computer work, take medications, and what you eat or drink can affect your sleep quality.

Tips to Eliminate Tossing and Turning

Why fight with sleep at night? If your mind is still wide awake long after your body has called it quits, there are steps you can take to promote sleep and prevent you from tossing and turning.

Reduce Alcohol Intake

If you drink alcohol, you'll notice that it acts as a sedative and aids sleep at first. But when you consume lots of alcohol over time, you might awaken in the middle of the night unable to sleep. That's because alcohol has a rebound effect later in the night. Prolonged dependency and addiction to alcohol disrupts sleep. And strong scientific evidence links alcoholism to insomnia.

Limit Nicotine and Caffeine

Lighting up and gulping down too much java, tea, or energy drinks can keep you up at night. Avoid nicotine and caffeine in the evenings before bedtime. They are stimulants and can keep you awake if you use them up to eight hours before bedtime.

Avoid Late-Night Meals

Eating late at night, especially eating heavy foods that are hard to digest, can keep you from nodding off. If you have to eat late, try lighter foods and avoid drinking too many fluids that can cause numerous trips to the bathroom.

Recharging Your Batteries

Ho hum. Some neuroscientists believe that yawning should be part of any stress reduction program and that you can yawn yourself to calm. Much like meditation, yawning lowers stress, puts you in a deep state of relaxation, and helps you drift off. Yawning acts like an air conditioner for your brain by putting more oxygen into your lungs and cooling down your neurological system. It's an emotional discharge that calms your body, sending the message that your system is powering down. So before your next stressful meeting, test, speech, or tossing and turning episode, yawn intentionally as many times as you can. If you have trouble getting started, fake it until you make it. You might feel silly at first. But once your stress drops and you're relaxed, the sandman will be there before you know it.

Forbid Electronic Devices in the Bedroom

Avoid working on your BlackBerry or iPad right up until bedtime. Texting or e-mailing late at night can overstimulate your brain, trigger adrenaline, and make it difficult for you to unwind. Also, try not to mentally solve problems or overthink a project at work after you've crawled into bed. A 2011 National Sleep Foundation study showed that the glow from electronic devices within an hour before bedtime suppresses melatonin and interferes with falling and staying asleep.

Stress Vocab

Melatonin is a hormone that promotes sleep and is naturally produced by the body.

Exercise Early in the Day

Exercising during the day releases stress, helps you fall asleep faster, and helps you sleep deeply through the night. But working out too close to bedtime can backfire on you. It can reenergize you and give you a second wind, making you feel like you're ready to embrace the day. As a rule, it's best to exercise earlier in the day or at least three to four hours before bedtime.

Put a Time Limit on Naps

If your sleep is fragmented at night, short day naps can make up the sleep debt and improve your mental performance. But napping for too long during the day can interfere with your nighttime sleep. If you do take naps, limit them to thirty minutes. Power napping earlier instead of later in the day can actually help you sleep better.

Power Napping

A Pew Research Center survey found that 34 percent of Americans take daily naps. I'm one of those who loves his midday snooze. It flips off my power switch and reboots my engine for the rest of the day. And I find that power napping far outweighs the benefits of chugging a Red Bull or drinking five cups of coffee to keep me alert and energized through the afternoon.

Stress Vocab

Power naps, commonly known as catnaps, are short midday naps of no more than thirty minutes.

Benefits of Power Naps

As part of his training regimen for the Tour de France race, cyclist Lance Armstrong napped during the day. President John Kennedy caught some extra z's in early afternoon to keep up his stride. And NASA pilots take in-flight naps to enhance performance and alertness.

Businesses have caught on because of the benefits of alertness, reduction in errors, and productivity. More companies are encouraging employees to take power naps at work. Some even provide special rooms with specially designed chairs for power napping.

Recharging Your Batteries

What the scientists tell us about the benefits of power napping match what I've noticed from my own naps. Studies at the Salk Institute show that the brain activity, memory, and mood of power nappers stays higher throughout the day compared to the brain activity of non-nappers, which declines as the day drags on. Another study conducted by the Harvard School of Public Health found that people who power nap were 34 percent less likely to die from heart problems.

Power naps are great stress buffers. They lower stress by reducing the level of cortisol in your blood, refreshing you and refueling your engine. My personal physician is a big advocate of power naps, and I usually take a fifteen-minute mid-afternoon nap on my office sofa between seeing clients. In fact, I just took one before writing on this topic. I always awaken feeling more energized and clearheaded. And the research on power napping bears out my personal experience. Here are some of the benefits:

➤ Improves brain function

➤ Boosts ability to process and store information

➤ Sharpens alertness, reducing the frequency of errors and accidents

➤ Increases productivity

➤ Elevates mood

➤ Lowers blood pressure and promotes healthy functioning of the heart

➤ Strengthens memory

Creating the Best Power Nap Ever

If you are interested in reducing your daily stress level, you might give the power nap a try. Midday napping is not for everyone, and some people have trouble sleeping during the daytime. But for many people, including myself, it's the best thing since sliced bread. The best time to power nap is around two or three o'clock in the afternoon. Here are some tips that I've found useful from my own power naps:

➤ Set an alarm: If you nap for more than fifteen to thirty minutes, you might fall into deep sleep and wake up with a headache, feel groggy, or have difficulty sleeping later that night.

➤ Minimize disruptions: Turn off your electronic devices and nap in a quiet place. I use ear plugs to ensure my full fifteen minutes of uninterrupted sleep.

➤ Limit caffeine: If you plan to power down after lunch, avoid drinking a lot of coffee or energy drinks earlier in the day. Caffeine can prevent you from falling asleep unless you drink it right before dosing off.

Shock Absorber

Consider taking a caffeine nap in the middle of the day if you're drowsy. Scientists say this is an effective strategy to achieve maximum alertness after a few winks. Have a caffeinated drink right before your power nap. After waking from a fifteen- or twenty-minute nap—the time it takes for your bloodstream to absorb the caffeine—you feel an energy burst from the double hit of caffeine and the power nap.

➤ Be comfortable: Although some people sleep with their heads on their desks or lying back in an office chair, I sprawl out on my office sofa and use the cushion for my head. Whatever your preference, make sure your supports are adequate and the room temperature is comfortable so that you can get to sleep right away.

➤ Darken the room: Too much light makes it difficult to power nap. I turn off the lights in my office and draw the blinds—both of which creates enough darkness for sleep. If you have limited options, keep a sleep mask in your desk drawer to block out excess light.

➤ Clear your mind: Make every effort to keep your power nap a stress-free zone. Free your mind of any thoughts, worries, or concerns, and tell yourself that this is your twenty or thirty minutes (and nobody else's). Remind yourself that you have the rest of the day to deal with other problems or unfinished business.

➤ Reboot gently: Some people wake from a power nap feeling sluggish, usually because they've slept too long. But if you feel disoriented, give yourself a few minutes to perk up. After my power nap, I rub my arms and thighs to feel myself back in my body and splash my face with cold water. Then I'm ready to embrace another few hours in the day.

Steps to Get to the Land of Nod

Before you hit the hay, familiarize yourself with some routines and other surefire steps you can take to catch more z's at night.

Regular Bedtime Hours

Go to bed around the same time every day and get up at the same time. Sticking to a routine (even on weekends) will keep your body regulated and make it easier for you to fall asleep. Use the if-then plan from Chapter 6 to develop healthier bedtime habits and routines.

If your goal is to get more sleep by going to bed earlier, your plan might look something like this: "When ten o'clock rolls around on weeknights, I'll hit the hay." You automatically recognize the "if" event, ten o'clock on a weeknight, which cues you to take the "then" action, go to bed.

Bedtime Conditions

Make sure your bedroom is cozy, inviting, and well ventilated. Be sure you have a comfortable, supportive mattress and pillow. Block out any light to create a dark room before you start counting sheep. Exposure to bright light within hours before sleep can trigger your brain to raise cortisol levels, creating a second wind, tricking your brain into thinking it's time to start instead of end your day.

Studies show that aircraft, road traffic, and railway noise, in that order, are common sounds that can interrupt sleep. If noise is a problem, try ear plugs to create a quieter sleep space.

Exclusive Use

Spending time in your bed for activities other than sleep and sex is a deal breaker. Go to bed only when you're sleepy. Use your bed exclusively for sleeping and sex, not for working on your laptop, arguing, eating, or watching TV. When you think of your bed and sleeping, you want to have positive associations.

Calming Routines

Avoid going to bed when your mind is racing with worry. Wait until you've calmed your mind and you're tired before you tuck yourself in. Have a consistent routine so that your body starts to anticipate sleep. Engage in calm activity to help your body power down, unwind, and get ready to drift off: a cup of hot chamomile tea, an inspirational book, a warm bath, soft soothing music, meditation, or muscle relaxation.

Recharging Your Batteries

According to researchers at the Group Health Research Institute, listening to soothing music while breathing deeply is just as beneficial as a massage for reducing stress. So if sleep won't come, find a softly lit place where you won't be distracted. Sit or lie down in a comfortable position. Then strap on your iPod and listen to soft instrumentals or recordings of nature sounds. Research shows that ten weekly hour-long sessions relieves symptoms of stress, worry, and depression. And the best part of all is that your body gets the deep rest it needs.

Dealing with Insomnia

Studies show that most people toss and turn because of work stress. Others can't sleep because of personal anxieties and worries. If you're still staring at the ceiling or eyeballing the clock twenty minutes after bedtime, get out of bed. The last thing you want to do is associate sleeplessness with your bed. When sleep won't come, go to another place in your house and practice one of the relaxation exercises from Chapters 10 and 11. Studies show that meditation and relaxation exercises improve slumber quality and length of sleep. Plus they reduce the number and frequency of nightmares. If you have chronic insomnia, consult your health care provider for the best sleep solutions for you.

"Rx from Dr. Bryan"

The Doctor Of Calm Is In

Sleep that knits up the raveled sleeve of care . . .

—William Shakespeare

When you get ready for bed, do you have a drowsy chaperone (worries that accompany you)? If so, imagine that you are leaving your cares at the office or in another room in your house. Instead of negative thoughts, conjure up positive images of your pet's loving eyes, your child's smiling face, or a fond memory that warms your heart. Think about all the treasures you're grateful for or practice a relaxation exercise. My prescription: Each night before bedtime, take a chill pill—instead of a sleeping pill— to relax your mind. As you put it at ease, let sleep mend your raveled sleeve, and you'll saw more logs than a lumberjack. Here's to outsmarting your stress!

Stress and Mind and Body Wellness

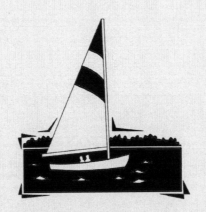

CHAPTER 9

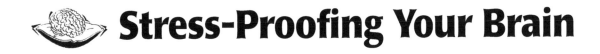 # Stress-Proofing Your Brain

In This Chapter

➤ How your brain works under stress

➤ Why your brain makes you sizzle

➤ Staying cool under pressure

➤ Rewiring your brain to put the brakes on stress

In this chapter, you'll discover the role your brain plays in everyday stress. You'll learn why, when trying to protect you, this coordinating hub of electrical activity sometimes causes you to flip out. You'll find tips on how to actually reengineer the way your brain responds to stress so you can stay cool under pressure. Plus, you'll discover what neuroscience says about the link between stress-resilience and spirituality.

Your Gray Matters: Get to Know it

If you're like most people, you might not even know about your own brain, and yet your brain is who you are. It is the boss of your mind and body. So it's important to know what it's up to, especially when you're feeling pressured. With modern imaging techniques, scientists have advanced our understanding of this amazing organ and how it functions under stress. You can refer to the figure, which shows the parts of the brain related to stress that I discuss in this chapter.

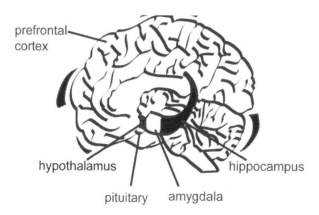

prefrontal
cortex

hypothalamus

hippocampus

pituitary   amygdala

Figure: *Side view of the human brain*

Stress Vocab

Neurons are brain cells that process and transmit messages through electrochemical impulses from one part of the brain to another.

Stress Vocab

The limbic system is buried beneath the cortex on top of the brain stem. It is a complex group of brain structures (including the amygdala, hypothalamus, and hippocampus) that are responsible for the formation of memories and emotions related to survival such as anxiety, fear, and anger.

Your brain is about the size of your fist and weighs about as much as a cantaloupe—around 3 pounds. Although it's mostly made up of water, the human brain contains as many as 100 billion neurons. These neurons connect through long, spidery arms, and communicate with each other through electrochemical signals. Your brain never shuts down; it's active even when you're asleep.

What Happens in Your Brain to Make You Sizzle?

Ever wonder why certain situations send you over the edge while others are a piece of cake for you to handle? Or why you hit the roof for something your spouse or partner says or does and then regret it after the damage is done? Studies in neuroscience explain what happens on a cellular level to spark those inner firestorms. We now know more about what upsets you, why it's difficult to control those hair-trigger reactions, and what you can do to prevent them.

Your Limbic System: Watch Your Step, Buddy

You might remember from earlier chapters that your brain (and mine) is wired to constantly scan your inner and outer worlds for threats and to react automatically to perceived threats. Emotional reactions come from the limbic system, sometimes called the reptilian brain or emotional brain. When this part of your brain registers situations as threatening, your stress response fires up.

Recharging Your Batteries

Are you waiting for the ax to fall or worrying that something bad might happen even though there's no good reason for it? If so, remind yourself that your limbic system is designed to exaggerate fears and worries for your protection. Then get curious and see if you can gain more clarity about why you're upset. Ask yourself questions like, "What am I afraid of?" "What are the chances of that really happening?" "What is the worst thing that could happen?" Curiosity, instead of anxiety is the gateway to clarity and calm. Plus, it kicks you into the executive function gear—your prefrontal cortex—creating an impartial and objective perspective on the stressful situation. So next time you're about to blast off, call on your brain's curiosity to help you stay on the launch pad.

Inside your brain, the hypothalamus sends emergency instructions to the rest of your body through the autonomic nervous system (ANS) discussed in Chapter 1. These messages cause your ANS to amp up salivation, sweating, heart rate, breathing, and digestion. That's when you feel your body reacting to the stress.

Your stress response might cause you to rant and rave, freeze in fear, or run away. Your limbic system doesn't have a sense of time or place. A threat is a threat. Much of the time, your brain's reaction in the present is driven by past events that are no longer deadly or unsafe. In other words, your brain and body overreact to small things that create unnecessary and unpleasant stress in the present moment—all in an effort to keep you safe.

Stress Vocab

The prefrontal cortex is the part of the brain located beneath your forehead in the frontal lobes. It is responsible for executive function, which allows you to reason logically, predict outcomes, judge right from wrong, and think rationally and abstractly.

Stress Vocab

The hypothalamus is the thermostat for your limbic system that controls balance in such bodily functions as hunger, thirst, sex, and response to pain. It regulates your autonomic nervous system and pituitary gland.

The pituitary gland is the part of your brain—controlled by the hypothalamus—that pumps stress hormones and endorphins into your bloodstream.

The Amygdala: Getting in Touch with Your Inner Reptile

Imagine peeking inside your own brain from a side view (check out the figure of the brain). The limbic system, or reptilian brain, houses old hurts from the past. Current events that trigger these reactions can be keys to ancient hurts—memories of past situations buried deep within your reptilian brain that angered, hurt, or scared you.

In the center of your limbic system, you'd spy a tiny almond-shaped gland called the amygdala. The amygdala contains a library of past feelings linked with past events. When your amygdala senses that present situations are similar to those already recorded by your reptilian brain, it kicks into survival mode to defend you. When your buttons get pushed, you can feel that moment when your amygdala dumps a tonic of heart-pounding enzymes into your bloodstream. The surging adrenaline and cortisol act like a tidal wave, hijacking your thoughts and leaving your emotions to rush to action.

Stress Vocab

Amygdala is an almond-shaped gland housed in your limbic system. It is a repository for memory and emotion and when triggered, it switches on emotional responses necessary for survival.

Your Amygdala and Relationships

Suppose you've had two heartbreaking romances. Chances are you would approach the third with a certain degree of trepidation. You might even avoid the third paramour because of a prediction in the library of your brain that the new relationship will also leave you with a broken heart.

Another way your amygdala shows up in relationships is when certain personalities remind you of someone who hurt you in the past. You might catch yourself automatically reacting to certain people with anger or harsh criticism, as if they were the actual ones who originally hurt you.

There's an old saying among neuroscientists: neurons that fire together, wire together. Carol is a case in point. When she and her husband stepped into the elevator of a fifth-floor restaurant to celebrate their tenth wedding anniversary, her heart catapulted to her throat and her stomach sank. The name of the hotel, emblazoned inside the elevator, hit her with the sudden memory that this was where her husband had had an affair one year earlier.

With lightning speed, Carol's stress response seared through her brain, dampening the celebration. Her amygdala rushed back all of the previous hurt and anger, which she unleashed on her startled husband who was confused by the outburst.

Shock Absorber

Here's an exercise to douse the firestorm when you get reactive: Recall any unpleasant reactions you've had in a previous relationship or situation. In your stress journal, make two columns labeled Present and Past. In the first column, jot down what you remember that made you sizzle because of past history. Then jot down the past experience in the second column. What does your blueprint from the past tell you about what is written in the "library books" housed in your amygdala? And what role, if any, do you think your amygdala might have played in these episodes?

Your Empathic Brain

Imagine having dinner with someone special in an expensive restaurant. You've looked forward to a quiet evening of candlelight, soft music, and intimate conversation. But your server is impatient and short-tempered. How would you feel? Most people would say annoyed or angry.

But then a friend seated at another table comes over to inform you that two of the server's three sons were killed in a car wreck the previous week. But she's a single mom and had to come to work. Now how would you feel? Most people would say, sad, sorry, or empathetic.

What happened? How can your emotions swing from anger one second to compassion the next? The server hasn't changed. Your perspective has changed because you have more information than you had to begin with. Now you see more of who the server really is. In neuroscience terms, your brain switched from firing a limbic system shot to lighting up your warm-hearted insula.

Stress Vocab

Insula is a receiving zone in your cerebral cortex—folded between the frontal and temporal lobes of the brain—that reads your body's internal states, fosters self-awareness, helps you attune to your inner sensations, and develops empathy for others.

Your brain routinely assesses risks by making judgments about people and situations. And negative experiences grab your brain's attention more than positive ones. Without your friend's insight, you probably would have continued to judge your server's behavior in a negative way.

Truth Serum

Brain scans show that your insula lights up when you practice mindfulness (see Chapter 12). When you are mindful of your breath and body sensations and bring deeper layers of feelings into your awareness, you activate the insula, which heightens compassion. Studies show that benevolent givers have brain scans that indicate better emotional health, heightened calm, less depression, and a greater sense of self-worth than the less compassionate. Perhaps science has given a whole new meaning to the old adage, It's better to give than to receive.

The Tend-and-Befriend Response to Stress

Both men and women react to stress with the aggressive fight-or-flight response. But scientists have discovered that many more women manage stress through the tending-and-befriending mode. In other words, they combat stress by nurturing their young (tending) and seeking togetherness by forming alliances through social support networks (befriending).

Examples of everyday tending and befriending might be attending a book club, talking on the phone with a close friend when you're upset, or asking for directions when you're lost. While both men and women secrete oxytocin during stress, the hormone's effects are neutralized in men by testosterone and other male hormones.

Both men and women have the biological fight-or-flight pattern of arousal (elevated heart rate and blood pressure). But men are more likely to react with fight (aggression) or flight (social withdrawal, substance abuse) in response to stress. Some scientists speculate that the six-year life expectancy difference between men and women can be explained by the male stress response putting men at greater health-related risks.

Stress Vocab

Oxytocin is a stress-reducing hormone secreted by the hypothalamus when you're threatened, damping the cortisol-induced fight-or-flight response and evoking a calm, relaxed mood.

Truth Serum

A team of researchers headed by Shelley Taylor at UCLA first identified the tend-and-befriend stress response. They found that touch activates this biologically based pattern, triggering the hormone oxytocin. Oxytocin is emitted by both men and women during stressful times. But contrary to the cortisol-mediated fight-or-flight response, oxytocin reduces fear and anxiety and neutralizes cortisol arousal associated with distress. It triggers softer emotions such as nurturing, caring, and social contact with others. Animals and people with a high level of oxytocin are calmer, more relaxed, and more socially engaged.

Beefing Up Your Prefrontal Cortex and Insula

If you want to be more alert, kinder, and more loving, you're in luck. Neuroimaging techniques show that stress diminishes activity in your prefrontal cortex and that long-term stress damages neurons, shrinks areas of your brain, and impairs thinking. On the flip side, brain scans at Harvard and UCLA show that through the regular practice of meditation, you can minimize brain shrinkage and cognitive decline, and build thicker neural tissues in the prefrontal cortex and insula.

Once beefed up, your gray matter sharpens attention, amps your immune system, neutralizes the amygdala's hotheaded reactions, heightens compassion, and shifts you into a calmer, kinder state of mind. I discuss the de-stressing benefits of meditation in Chapter 13.

Rewiring Your Brain to Stay Cool Under Pressure

Over time, your brain's perceived threat to repetitive stress can result in chronic mental and physical problems. Whether you're a harried parent, driven businessperson, or worried retiree coping with an uncertain future, these stressors eventually catch up with you. They force your brain to adapt negatively to them as only it can.

Truth Serum

Scientists at the National Institute of Mental Health report that the brain has the ability to change its wiring and grow new neural connections through regular practice and repetition of tasks. In other words, you have an innate ability to de-stress your brain by changing old practices of managing stress to new ones. The new practices reshape nerve cells and change the way your brain works.

But there's good news. This same process of negative adaptation can be used to heal as well as to harm. Did you know that you can reengineer your brain to calm your knee-jerk reactions. Sound like frontier science fiction? Hold on. Don't laugh in my face. I know it sounds far-fetched, but I'm not off my rocker.

The brain is prewired to be pliable just like a cut on your hand regenerates new healing tissue. This pliability is called neuroplasticity, and it allows you to use your mind to change the structure and functioning of your brain, no matter how old you are. Some experts go so far as to say it would take less than two months for you to alter your neural functioning.

Stress Vocab

Neuroplasticity is the pliability of the brain that makes it possible to rewire its connection of neurons to adapt to stressful conditions in the external world.

Remember that old saying? When cells fire together, they wire together. By taking a different tack under pressure, you can wire stressful events with a more positive action and get a calmer consequence. With some dedication to changing your old stress responses, you change the way your brain is firing in the moment. So when you do something different, the firing of neural pathways wires the different approach and its outcome.

Override Your Reptilian Brain's Threats

When you're frazzled, you can avoid hotheaded action and cool down your amygdala by challenging perceived threats. Here are some examples of how to do that:

➤ Try to see the upside of downside situations—to see the roses instead of the thorns: "I have to pay more taxes this year than ever before" becomes "I made more money this year than I've ever made."

➤ Be chancy and take small risks in new situations instead of predicting negative outcomes without sticking your neck out: "I won't go to the party because I'm afraid I won't know anyone" becomes "If I go to the party, I might have a chance to make new friends."

➤ Make an effort to focus on the good news wrapped around the bad news: "My neighbor's house was destroyed by the tornado" becomes "Their house is gone, but everyone survived and nobody was injured."

➤ Avoid blowing things out of proportion and letting one negative experience rule your whole life pattern: "I didn't get the promotion, so now I'll never reach my career goals" becomes "I didn't get the promotion, but there are many more steps I can take to reach my career goals."

Rewind the Mini-Movies Playing in Your Head

In his book *Buddha's Brain : The Practical Neuroscience of Happiness, Love, and Wisdom,* neuropsychologist Rick Hanson describes what he calls mini-movies. Think of your brain as a simulator constantly running mini-movies—brief clips that are building blocks of conscious mental activity. These mini-movies of past or possible future events at one time wired people for survival by strengthening the brain's ability to learn successful behaviors through repeated neural firing patterns.

Today, because of your genetic heritage, your brain continues to produce short movie clips that have nothing to do with survival or with what's happening in the present. But even if you know that, it's easy to get caught up in the storyline and stress yourself out in the heat of the moment.

When the clips play, they can pull you out of the present and create stressful thoughts and feelings. You might fret about a lost love, agonize about an unreachable goal, or rehearse for a challenging presentation at work. Your mini-movies can become bars on an invisible cage that trap you in a life smaller than the one you could actually have—much like a tiger released into a large park but continues to crouch as if it's still confined in its old pen.

Recharging Your Batteries

You can untangle yourself from your mind's miniseries by simply paying attention to when old movies pop up, eclipsing the present situation as it really is. Remind yourself that your brain is wired this way. When you start to sizzle, instead of automatically reacting, ask yourself what old, familiar feelings the experience is bringing up. Usually, you'll realize that it's an inner movie reel, not the present person or circumstance. Gently bring your wandering mind back to connect with the present moment and engage your prefrontal cortex.

Check In with Your Prefrontal Cortex

Another way to change your brain's wiring is to get in the habit of engaging your prefrontal cortex when stress blindsides you. Your prefrontal cortex gives you the capacity to take a breath, step back, and regain an outsider's perspective in the midst of threats.

Next time you're pressed, go inside and focus on your inner experience. Acknowledge and listen to your feelings. Then ask, "What am I feeling in my body right now? What are the feelings telling me? If my heart wasn't slamming against my chest, what would I do right now?" When you're under pressure and engage the executive function of your prefrontal cortex, it's easier to separate from automatic limbic reactions, stay cool, and make smarter decisions.

When I realize my limbic system is activated, I check in with myself and ask if I'm angry, upset, or worried. I acknowledge those feelings as parts of myself. Then, I dialogue with those feelings: "I know you're upset. How can I help?" This gives me immediate separation from the reactions, throws the switch in the executive function of my brain, and enables me to act instead of react.

Another strategy to activate your prefrontal cortex to keep you from going into orbit is to trump your amygdala with the acronym WAIT:

Watch for activated parts of you that are triggered by a stressful situation. Once you notice the activation,

Avoid your usual reaction and imagine stepping back and taking a breath.

Invite the activated feeling to relax, and, with curiosity and compassion, soothe it so it calms down, allowing you to act instead of react.

Turn each stress reaction into an opportunity to calm yourself, and then act until you undo the old habit.

Activating Your Parasympathetic Nervous System

As I mentioned earlier, your ANS plays a starring role in your emotional life when it is engaged by your hypothalamus. Usually, you're not aware of your ANS except when you're stressed out and it revs up your body functions. Your ANS is composed of two parts: the sympathetic nervous system (SNS) and the parasympathetic nervous system (PNS). The SNS activates your body functions during stressful emergencies to help you get away.

Stress Vocab

The sympathetic nervous system (SNS) is a part of your autonomic nervous system that functions in opposition to the parasympathetic nervous system by mobilizing your body's defense systems to induce your stress response for survival.

The parasympathetic nervous system (PNS) is a part of your autonomic nervous system that functions in opposition to the sympathetic nervous system by calming your body's defense systems to induce your rest and digest response.

Your Rest and Digest Response

Your (PNS) dampens down your body functions in nonemergencies, allowing you to rest and digest. Although you need both systems, your SNS and PNS work in opposition to each other. Think of your SNS as the gas. It dilates your pupils, increases your heart rate, opens bronchial tubes in your lungs, and inhibits secretions in your digestive system. In contrast, your PNS is the brakes. It constricts your pupils, decreases your heart rate, constricts your bronchial tubes and slows breathing, and stimulates activity in your stomach and intestines.

Both systems are vital for life. Bringing a balance between the two is the holy grail of stress management. When your SNS trumps your PNS to the point that your mental and physical health are at stake, you can activate your rest and digest response.

First off, ask yourself how much time you devote to your PNS to keep your mind and body in harmony. If you're like many harried people nowadays, your answer would be "not enough." You can switch on your PNS and put the brakes on your SNS by engaging in certain activities such as exercising briskly, yawning, relaxing in nature, taking power naps, and the following practices, which I discuss in future chapters: practicing deep breathing, yoga, tai chi, and progressive muscle relaxation; praying; meditating; laughing; and getting a massage.

Truth Serum

Studies show that you can stress-proof your brain through calming activities and spiritual practices. Brain scans demonstrate that contemplating of nature, meditating, and praying activate your brain's frontal lobes (behind the forehead) and reduce activity in the parietal lobes at the top rear of your head. These changes heighten dopamine and dampen epinephrine squirts in your brain. Neuroscientists say these neurological changes create a feeling of calm, unity, transcendence, and a feeling of unification with God or consciousness. The poet Emily Dickinson might have been on to something when she said, "The brain is just the weight of God."

Stress Vocab

Dopamine is a neurotransmitter released in the brain that creates feelings of euphoria and well-being.

Creating Rest and Digest Under Pressure: A Fable

A Chinese farmer had a horse for tilling his fields, his most valuable possession. One day the horse escaped into the hills, and the farmer's neighbors sympathized with him: "What bad luck you have." But the farmer replied, "Bad luck? Good luck? Who knows? A week later the horse returned with a herd of wild horses from the hills. This time the neighbors congratulated the old man on his good luck. His reply again was, "Good luck? Bad luck? Who knows?

Later when the farmer's son was attempting to tame one of the wild horses, he fell off its back and broke his leg. The neighbors shook their heads in sympathy, again saying, "What bad luck you have." But the farmer's only reply was, "Bad luck? Good luck? Who knows?" Weeks later, the army marched into the village and conscripted every able-bodied man they could find to fight in a bloody war. When they saw the farmer's son with his broken leg, they let him off. Now, was that bad luck or good luck?

The farmer was a wise man, taking a calm, neutral stand instead of reacting to life's ups and downs. You might say his PNS overrode his amygdala. You could also say that his alarmed neighbors let their SNS hijack them into an emotional roller-coaster ride. They overestimated the perceived threats instead of looking for the possibility that each "bad" outcome might have something good wrapped around it.

It's a No-Brainer

Even when positive experiences outnumber negative ones, it can feel like your life is full of mostly negative experiences. That can make you feel on edge, pessimistic, and grim. The key is to look for the silver lining in unpleasant situations and to note and savor positive outcomes so you have a balanced perspective.

Once you realize things are usually not as bad as your brain registers them to be, you can take a breath, step back from unnerving events, and, hopefully, relax. You don't have to look through rose-colored glasses, but don't look at your plight as hopeless or overwhelming, either. By deliberately bringing a different part of your brain (your PNS) to threatening situations, you can create a more peaceful life inside and out.

The Doctor Of Calm Is In

Your brain . . . [is] like Velcro for negative experiences and Teflon for positive ones

—Rick Hanson

By now, you might be dehydrated because the brain can be a pretty dry subject. My prescription: Inoculate yourself with a brain booster. Read the story of the farmer once or twice daily as needed or until your overreaction to stress subsides. And drink plenty of water. Here's to outsmarting your stress!

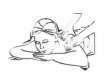

CHAPTER 10

Relaxing Your Body and Physical Wellness

In This Chapter

➤ Paying attention to your body

➤ How to use your breath to relax

➤ Using your body for tension reduction

➤ Types of body-calming techniques

In this chapter you'll discover how to change old habits and develop new physical measures to manage stress. You will become more aware of your body and learn to listen to it. Using techniques such as progressive muscle relaxation, breath awareness, stretching exercises, and massage you will have the tools you need to release tension, relax your body, and create physical wellness.

Listen to Your Body Talk

In her famous song, "Physical," Olivia Newton-John serenades, "Let me hear your body talk." And that's what this chapter is about: listening to your body speak to you, the body that has housed you for years. Chances are you don't pay much attention when it has something to say. If you're like most people, you've become so accustomed to living in your body that you're not aware when it speaks to you.

Most of the tools needed for inducing relaxation and physical wellness are right within you. By using the physical apparatus you already have—your muscles, breath, and attention—you become more aware of what's going on in your body. This will allow you to change old habits and develop more effective ones for decreasing your stress. Let's start with a body inventory.

Recharging Your Batteries

The pendulum exercise refers to the natural swing of your nervous system between sensations of well-being and stress or tension. This exercise brings your attention to the presence of natural relaxation that can get eclipsed by stressful body sensations.

With your eyes closed, notice a place in your body where you feel stress or choose an area from your checklist. It can show up as pain, tension, an ache, or constriction. Then swing your attention to a place in your body where you feel less stress or no stress. Focus there on the absence of stress, noticing your body sensations: steady heartbeat, slowed breathing, warmed skin, softened jaw, loose muscles. Remain focused there and note the sensation. Then imagine that sensation spreading to other parts of your body.

Now shift back to the place where you originally felt stress. If it has changed, pay attention to the change. Continue moving your attention back and forth between what is left of the stress and the relaxed parts of your body. As you shift, note where stress is lessening and spend some time paying attention to the lessening so that it can spread to other parts of your body.

Inventory Your Body as It Speaks to You

Chances are you're not aware of the stress that builds up from day to day. Maybe you keep plugging away, ignoring the stiffness and soreness that your body stores. A body scan lets you take an inventory of the areas holding stress that you might not even be aware of.

Find a quiet place where you can sit or lie flat comfortably and relax as much as you can. Then slowly start scanning at your feet, working your way up your body muscle by muscle. As you move up, focus on each muscle group one at a time. Note areas where you're holding tension, tightness, or pain or places that are stiff, sore, or sensitive without labeling the sensations good or bad.

You don't have to do anything about the discomfort yet; just notice for now. The goal here is to take an inventory as your body talks to you. We'll get into the tension relief later. For now, just notice the tense areas and bring all of your attention to each spot, focusing there for about fifteen seconds. Again, there's nothing to do except pay attention.

Your Personal Relaxation Checklist

After you've finished with your body inventory, make a personal relaxation checklist in your stress journal of all the places where you're holding stress. You might notice strained shoulders, lower back soreness, tiredness behind your eyes, stiffness in the right side of your neck, rigid jaw, or tightness in your hamstrings. As you read on, I'll show you many variations on how to relax those places that you might identify in your checklist.

Progressive Muscle Relaxation

One of the quickest and easiest ways to drain tension is through a practice called progressive muscle relaxation (PMR). PMR helps you become more aware of muscle tension, where you hold it in your body, and how muscle tension feels different from muscle relaxation.

PMR was built on the premise that since muscle tension accompanies stress, muscle relaxation can reduce stress. The goal is to develop a state of deep relaxation by gradually releasing stress that you're holding in different muscles of your body by progressing from one muscle group to the next.

The idea is to tense a muscle

Stress Vocab

Progressive muscle relaxation is a technique for reducing stress and creating a state of deep relaxation by moving attention from one muscle group to the next, alternately tensing and relaxing the muscles.

Truth Serum

Developed by Dr. Edmund Jacobson in the 1920s, progressive muscle relaxation has all the benefits of the relaxation response (discussed in the next chapter). Studies show that PMR, when practiced fifteen to twenty minutes daily for a month or two, can improve concentration, reduce anxiety, lower blood pressure, and promote overall physical health.

for ten seconds while noticing how the tension feels. Then you relax the muscle for twenty seconds, noticing how the relaxation feels. This technique helps you gain a sense of how different tension and relaxation feel.

Steps to Progressive Muscle Relaxation

As you begin to progress to different muscle groups, be careful to tighten, not strain, your muscles. Apply a firm tension to each muscle but don't create pain, over-exertion, or undue discomfort. Keep your mind focused on the muscle you are tensing. When your mind wanders, gently bring it back and focus on that muscle again. Remember, when you tense a muscle for ten seconds, pay attention to how the tension feels. As you relax the muscle, savor that feeling for twenty seconds, letting it deepen. Here are the steps that you can practice:

➤ Sit or lie in a quiet location where you won't be distracted. Wear loose clothing, and make sure cell phones, children, and pets are out of earshot. Scan your body, noticing which muscles are tense and which ones are relaxed.

➤ Start by clenching both fists and tightening your forearms for about ten seconds. Notice how the muscles in your hands and forearms feel while they're tensed. Then release the tension in your hands and arms. As they relax, take about twenty seconds and pay attention to how that feels.

➤ Next, draw your arms up, bending your elbows so that your hands are touching your shoulders, tightening both of your biceps. Hold for ten seconds and notice the feeling of tension, then release for twenty seconds and notice the feeling of relaxation.

➤ Extend your arms straight out and lock your elbows. Tense your triceps, the muscles on the underside of your upper arms. Hold and notice for ten seconds, then loosen and notice for 20 seconds.

➤ Scrunch up your facial muscles. Tighten your forehead and wrinkle your nose. Squint your eyelids shut, purse your lips, and bite down on your teeth. Hold and notice for ten seconds, then loosen and notice for twenty seconds.

➤ Form your mouth into a large zero, opening your jaws as wide as you can. Hold and notice for ten seconds, then let your jaw hang limp and notice for twenty seconds.

➤ Tighten the muscles in the back of your neck by extending your neck gently backward toward your spine. Remember to avoid straining yourself. Hold and notice for ten seconds, then release and notice for twenty seconds.

➤ Gently drop your chin toward your chest. Hold and notice for ten seconds, then release and notice for twenty seconds.

➤ Tilt your head gently to your left shoulder, feeling the tension in the right side of your neck. Hold and notice for ten seconds, then release and notice for twenty seconds. Then do the same movement but tilt your head to your right shoulder, holding and noticing for ten seconds and releasing and noticing for twenty seconds.

> ➤ Raise both shoulders toward your ears. Hold them tightly and notice for ten seconds, then let your shoulders fall limp and notice for twenty seconds.

> ➤ Press your shoulders back, bringing shoulder blades as close together as you can. Hold and notice for ten seconds, then loosen and notice for twenty seconds.

> ➤ Suck in your stomach muscles and arch your back (gently please). Skip this part of the exercise if you have any type of back problem. Hold and notice for ten seconds, then release and notice for twenty seconds.

> ➤ Extend your legs, squeezing the muscles in your thighs and hips and tightening your calf muscles. Point your toes toward your head. Hold and notice for ten seconds, then release and notice for twenty seconds.

> ➤ Do a brief body scan starting at the crown of your head and working your way down to your toes, paying attention to what you're feeling in your body. Focus your attention on any muscle group that feels tense. Imagine the relaxation from adjacent areas of your body spreading into those tense areas. Take about sixty seconds to sit or lie quietly while you savor the relaxed feeling in your body. You can imagine yourself floating or in a pleasant place.

Don't Just Do Something, Sit There!

By now, you might be shaking your head thinking, "There's no way I'll ever take the time to practice muscle relaxation." But time off from your active regimen—whether from strenuous exercise or a stressful schedule—is just as important as the regimen itself. Total relaxation reduces the level of stress hormones, promotes a greater storage of glycogen in the muscles, and reduces muscular tension. Plus, it activates your parasympathetic nervous system, the part of your autonomic nervous system (discussed in Chapter 9) that soothes and calms you.

Recharging Your Batteries

Think of yourself as a bank account. If stress is withdrawing more than relaxation is depositing, you could be headed for bankruptcy (burnout). Setting aside fifteen minutes to an hour a day to practice either the pendulum, progressive muscle relaxation, or deep breathing exercise can keep you "open for business." Think of it as building your personal investments so that your daily deposits equal the withdrawals that stress makes from your account.

Breath Awareness and Relaxation

Breathing is something you probably take for granted because it's automatic and you've been doing it since the day you were born. But right under your nose is a valuable antidote to stress: your breath.

When Stress Steals Your Breath Away

Your spouse or partner is suffocating you with impossible demands. A coworker is taking the wind out of your sails. Your boss is breathing down your neck. An emergency call from a family member causes you to hold your breath. You are on the verge of a meltdown.

Chances are when you're freaking out, you overbreathe. Your breath becomes short, shallow, and rapid. You use your shoulders instead of your diaphragm to move air in and out of your lungs. You might even stop breathing or hold your breath and not even realize it. Overbreathing (or hyperventilating) expels too much carbon dioxide from the bloodstream and upsets your body's balance of gases, increasing your stress level.

Stress Vocab

The diaphragm is the muscle housed between your abdominal cavity and your chest cavity that helps you with deep breathing.

This is in direct contrast to what happens when you're calm and relaxed: your breathing is slower, fuller, and deeper, coming from your abdomen. When you breathe from your abdomen, your diaphragm flattens downward, pushing the muscles in the abdominal cavity upward, creating more space in the chest so that your lungs can fill up. You can't get as worked up if you force yourself to breathe deeply. Your body can't maintain the same level of stress with the extra oxygen you get in your bloodstream when you breathe from your abdomen.

Shock Absorber

The acronym HALT stands for hungry, angry, lonely, or tired. It is a gentle reminder for you to stop and breathe deeply when stress overtakes you. You can switch off your stress response when you intentionally breathe with your diaphragm. Take a deep abdominal breath through your nose, holding it as you count slowly to six. Purse your lips and exhale slowly through them. Repeat this breathing pattern several times, relaxing your body further with each breath. Next time things become too much for you, remember to HALT, take a few deep abdominal breaths through your nose, and you might not have to blow your top.

Natural Abdominal Breathing

Deep breathing from your abdomen sends additional oxygen to your brain and activates your parasympathetic nervous system, which creates a calming, soothing effect throughout your body. Notice how you're breathing right now. Do your breaths come from high in your chest or deep in your abdomen? Are they fast or slow? If you are aware of shallow breathing patterns, higher up in your chest, you can calm yourself by practicing abdominal or diaphragmatic breathing. It's difficult to hold on to stress and relax at the same time.

Steps to Natural Abdominal Breathing

When you breathe naturally, the way you did as a newborn, your abdomen expands as you inhale, and it contracts as you exhale. By practicing natural abdominal breathing, you can achieve a state of deep relaxation. And it only takes five minutes. Here's how it works:

➤ Place one hand on your chest, the other on your belly.

➤ Keeping your upper chest still, gently and slowly inhale a normal amount of air through your nose, and slowly count to four on the inbreathe. As you bring the air into the lowest part of your lungs, notice your abdomen rise on the inbreathe and fall on the outbreathe. Your chest should barely move in abdominal breathing.

➤ After each inhale, hold your breath briefly, then exhale slowly and gently, again counting to four, letting your entire body go limp.

➤ Repeat these steps for five minutes each day or do several five-minute sets per day. In a short while, you'll notice a big reduction in your stress level. Practice makes perfect, as the old saying goes. So the more you take the time to practice, the more moments of calm you will have, and your ability to relax will increase over time.

Recharging Your Batteries

I would be remiss if I didn't mention another essential ingredient besides *doing*: the special joy that comes from total relaxation through *being*. "Who the heck has time to waste sitting and watching the grass grow?" you might ask. To that I say that sacrificing your well-being to keep routines afloat is living as if *doing* is more important than *being*.

Schedule a hole in your calendar for unplanned moments, when there's nowhere to go, nothing to do, nobody to see. Create quiet reflective moments, where your mind can drift, your body can melt, and, yes, where you can watch the grass grow. Or lose yourself in a calming view of nature, kick a ball along the seashore, sip tea by a warm fire while stroking a pet, have a heart-to-heart talk with someone close to you. These soothing moments are the building blocks to well-being and being well.

Calming Breath Counts

Counting your breaths adds the extra dimension of concentration. This concentration introduces you to important aspects of meditation:

➤ Focusing on your breath

➤ Blocking intrusive thoughts

➤ Relaxing

➤ Centering yourself

This form of meditative breathing also has many of the same benefits as the relaxation response, which I discuss in the next chapter.

➤ In a quiet, comfortable place, close your eyes and focus on your breathing. Take a long, deep breath through your nostrils. Then slowly exhale.

➤ Take five easy breaths through your nose, imagining you are taking the air first into the bottom of your lungs, then moving into your upper lungs. On your inbreathe, pause for about five seconds. On your outbreathe, start counting down from five. It would look something like this:
Inhale, pause, exhale, "5"
Inhale, pause, exhale, "4"
Inhale, pause, exhale, "3"
Inhale, pause, exhale, "2"
Inhale, pause, exhale, "1"

➤ After your fifth outbreathe, start counting down from five again.

➤ After you've completed a few sets, open your eyes and stretch slightly.

➤ Keep your focus on counting with slow, easy breaths, letting your breathing find its own rhythm. If you lose count, no worries; just start over from the beginning. When stray thoughts come, just acknowledge them, let them go, and come back to counting your breaths.

Once you are comfortable with counting down from 5, you can practice counting backward from 10. But don't get hooked on the number. What's more important is your clear concentration. For best results, practice calming breath counts for fifteen to twenty minutes once or twice a day.

Truth Serum

Neuro-feedback—also known as biofeedback—is used to treat emotional and behavioral stress. Sensors are attached with a surgical paste to your scalp. These sensors allow the clinician to directly observe your brain waves. Those brain waves are then transformed into visual images on a game computer. You learn to make changes in the game's display by playing a simple video game and these changes create improvements in your nervous system.

Such changes can reduce your stress symptoms within hours or even minutes. Neuro-feedback is noninvasive to the body, and no chemical or electrical impulse enters your body. It's the learning from practice that enables you to regulate your nervous system, relax your body, and calm yourself. You can go online to find a neuro-feedback provider near you.

Stretching Your Tension Away

Stretching releases the stress that builds up in your body during the day. Even cats, dogs, and many other animals naturally stretch to discharge tension. Not only does it feel good, but stretching your body is one of the easiest and cheapest ways to reduce muscle tension and relax your body. Some other benefits of stretching include:

> ➤ Improved blood flow to your muscles

> ➤ Increased flexibility

> ➤ Enhanced sleep

> ➤ Sharpened mental alertness

> ➤ Improved posture

> ➤ Improved range of motion in your joints

Loosening Your Stress Triangle

The most common area of the body where people hold stress is in the stress triangle, the top of your shoulders and back of your neck. During stress, your shoulders lift up towards your ears in a shrug. If you notice this unconscious habit, as I often do, you can try the following stretch at home or in your office:

➤ Sitting or standing, lower your right ear to your right shoulder. Hold for ten seconds.

➤ Continue by reaching your left arm away from your body. Hold for ten seconds.

➤ Then reach your right arm to the left side of your forehead and gently pull the stretch a little further. Hold for the final thirty seconds.

➤ Release everything slowly in the reverse order and repeat on your left side.

Chest and Arm Stretch

You might have noticed that your chest muscles and the muscles in the front of your underarm are often tight from repeatedly reaching your arms out in front of your body. Typing on the computer, driving, holding a book, or working at your desk are activities that shorten these muscles after a long time. Here's a simple stretch for these muscles:

➤ Stand in a doorframe at the end of a wall with the front of your right shoulder pressing against the end of the wall. Reach your right hand directly out from your shoulder down the wall. Your hand and arm should be touching the wall, parallel to the floor.

➤ Begin to turn your body away from your right arm and feel the stretch.

➤ Repeat the same pattern with your left arm on the other side of the doorjamb, taking the turn a little further to gradually increase the stretch. You might feel your shoulder blade move closer to your spine when doing this stretch.

Hamstring Stretch

When you're in a seated position, your hamstrings are in a shortened or contracted state. So if you sit a lot or if you have sore muscles in your lower back from bending to clean or garden or from lifting packages or moving heavy objects, you'll find this stretch beneficial. Give this hamstring stretch a try as long as you don't have a lower back injury. To get started, you'll need to find a wall or a door opening.

Lie on your back with one leg stretched out on the floor, and press the other leg up against the wall reaching toward the ceiling. If your hamstrings are very tight (like mine are), you might need to move your hips further from the wall to start. Concentrate on keeping your knee straight but not locked. To increase the stretch, move your hips closer to the wall as you exhale. Doing so, your leg reaches further up the wall. Remember to relax every other part of your body. Repeat the same movements with the other leg.

After a long-term consistent routine of hamstring stretching combined with core strengthening exercises, you can become taller! I'm working on going from Danny DeVito (who is 4 feet 9.5 inches tall) to Clint Eastwood (who is 6 feet 4 inches tall). Stay tuned. I'll let you know how it goes.

Give the Fingers to Your Overstressed Body

Massage therapy is another method for relaxing your body and releasing muscle tension. Studies show that it lowers blood pressure, relieves pain and stiffness, reduces stress, and bumps up your immune system. In one study, people who received a forty-five minute Swedish massage had an 18 percent spike in infection-fighting white blood cells.

Types of Massage

Although there are many types of massage, Swedish massage is the most common. Shiatsu, or acupressure, is another popular type in which the therapist kneads pressure points in the body. A more aggressive approach, deep tissue massage, loosens stubborn knots that keep muscles tight and tense. I had a Thai massage in Thailand in which the masseuse straddled my back and used her fists to pound out stress, and her fingers, knuckles, and elbows to knead deep tissue. She braced her feet against my back and pulled my arms and legs to stretch the stress out of deep tissue. Although Thai massages leave me on cloud nine, I wouldn't recommend them for anyone with chronic pain, unable to tolerate deep tissue massage, or sensitive to the masseuse being up close and personal.

Recharging Your Batteries

Acupuncture, a procedure of inserting and manipulating thin needles into strategic points on the body to relieve pain, originated in China over 2,500 years ago. Scientists still haven't conducted enough studies to determine its effectiveness. But proponents say acupuncture boosts the body's natural painkillers and aids in blood flow. And some research shows that the procedure reduces nausea and vomiting after surgery and chemotherapy. Still, more research is needed to pinpoint (no pun intended) acupuncture's role in stress and pain reduction.

You can find an acupuncturist in your area by going online. If you decide to use this method of treatment, make sure your acupuncturist is well trained and endorsed by the appropriate state licensing unit if your state has one.

Professional Massage: The Magic Touch

If you've never had a professional massage, there's nothing like it. The exhilarating relief you get from a licensed massage therapist is a great way to soothe aches and pains and calm down after a hectic schedule. And if you tell the therapist where your discomfort resides, most can recommend the type of massage you need and find the tender spots in your body right away.

You are treated while lying on a massage table, sitting in a massage chair, or lying on a mat on the floor. Typically, you are unclothed with sheets or towels covering most of your body. The therapist uses a variety of heated oils such as coconut oil, lavender oil, grape seed oil, olive oil, almond oil, or mustard oil. The massager rubs the oils over your body using fingers, palms, and elbows to stimulate sore areas. Sometimes heated stones are used to penetrate warmth into stiff and tender tissue for loosening and tension release.

Self-Massage: Let Your Fingers Do the Walking

If visiting a massage therapist is not in the cards for you, here are some massage techniques from Northwestern Health Sciences University that you can try on yourself at your desk, in bed before falling asleep, or pretty much anywhere, anytime:

➤ Head: Using your fingertips, gently massage the area around your temples, forehead, and ears. Press your thumbs lightly into the area at the base of your skull.

➤ Scalp: Place your thumbs behind your ears while spreading your fingers on top of your head. Move your scalp back and forth slightly by making circles with your fingertips for fifteen to twenty seconds.

➤ Eyes: Close your eyes and place your ring fingers directly under your eyebrows near the bridge of your nose. Slowly increase the pressure for five to ten seconds, then gently release. Repeat two to three times.

➤ Sinuses: Place your fingertips at the bridge of your nose. Slowly slide your fingers down your nose and across the top of your cheekbones to the outside of your eyes.

➤ Neck: Using both of your thumbs, find the indentation where your neck meets your shoulders. Gently press your thumbs into the indentation and rub slowly.

➤ Shoulders: Reach one arm across the front of your body to your opposite shoulder. Using a circular motion, press firmly on the muscle above your shoulder blade. Repeat on the other side.

The Sweetness of Doing Nothing

All the physical relaxation in the world won't help you fully relax until you have mastered the art of passive rest. The Italians have a name for it: *il dolce far niente,* "the sweetness of doing nothing." It doesn't translate in the United States, where tasks and schedules define us. The closest phrase we have is *killing time.* But *il dolce far niente* demands more from you: that you intentionally let go and make *being* a priority. Not long ago, I noticed a man, arms out to his side, balancing on an old sea wall. In that moment, with all the time in the world and no hurry to get anywhere, all he cared about was navigating his body against the warm ocean breeze.

The Doctor Of Calm Is In

Passive rest has been compared with the pauses that are an intricate part of a beautiful piece of music....These absences of sound are what define the music. Without them, it would be just noise.

—Joe Friel, author of *Cycling Past Fifty*

My prescription: You, too, can find this sweetness of being alive by spending time without a goal—doing something for nothing more than the sheer pleasure of it. Indulge yourself with as many dosages of "sweet nothings" as often as needed for stress reduction or until stress symptoms subside. Here's to outsmarting your stress!

CHAPTER 11

Calming Your Mind and Restorative Rest

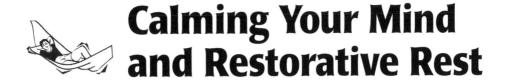

In this chapter, you'll discover the restorative properties of mental techniques and the effectiveness of using them together with physical relaxation. You'll find ways to slow down and relax your mind so that you feel less stressed and more productive. The soothing mental techniques presented here can undo what stress does to you on a daily basis and promote inner calm and overall emotional wellness.

Hit Your Pause Button

Talk show host Joy Behar said, "I don't like to relax; it stresses me out." And she is not alone. Many people say they have trouble sitting still. You too may be among the ranks of those who can't seem to quiet their minds. But relaxation is just as important to your mental and physical health as turning off your car engine once in a while to keep it from overheating. Studies show that calming your mind with doses of relaxation can be the best antidote to stress.

If your life is like that of most people, it demands that you stay busy and connected. You might even think that if you have a lot going on that you are living your life fully. That's certainly what today's culture would have you believe: the more the merrier. But the science of rest presents an opposing view.

Stress Vocab

Restorative rest is a state of mind similar to a waking sleep in which you feel a deep relaxation, slowed heartbeat and breathing, and reduced oxygen consumption.

Restorative Rest

The truth is that you're more alive when you are at peace with yourself, when you have a mind that's resting. A rested mind is a mind without imperative—one in which you don't need things to be different. You can relax and enjoy things just as they are without the urge to get rid of something, to stay busy, or to try to get something. I'm talking here about passive rest, not exertion like hiking, a game of tennis, or jogging with your iPod. That's recreation, not rest. Restorative rest includes activities in which you're not exerting yourself, thinking, or analyzing. It takes you out of the fight-or-flight mode, where you're under the gun to make a decision or get something done.

Truth Serum

If you make a decision when you're frustrated in a traffic jam or after a hard day's work, chances are it'll be different from one you'd make after a restful night's sleep. Why? Scientists have discovered a phenomenon known as decision fatigue—your brain is worn out, depleted of mental energy. After a day-long string of making ordinary decisions—such as what to wear, where to eat, how much to spend, when to agree or disagree at work—your mind gets fatigued. You're short with coworkers and loved ones; you eat junk food instead of your regular healthy meal; you permit your newly licensed teenager to drive the car on an icy night.

The more choices you make throughout the day, the harder each one becomes for your strained mind. So you start to take shortcuts by making impulsive decisions or by doing nothing. Although avoiding decisions eases your mental strain in the short term, it's more risky in the long run. The solution? Rest. Your mind needs restorative rest just like your body does when you're tired.

Mind-Calming Activities

This resting state stimulates your parasympathetic nervous system (see Chapter 9), healing your body from the wear and tear of everyday stress. The next time you're uptight, try one of the following mind-calming activities to unwind and clear your head:

➤ Immerse yourself in inspirational reading

➤ Soak in a warm bath or take a dip in a hot tub

➤ Sit by a warm fire and watch the flames

➤ Sit on the beach and feel the ocean breeze

➤ Engage in a fun hobby or craft

➤ Write in your stress journal

➤ Walk barefoot in a summer rain shower

➤ Take short nature walks without a goal

➤ Meditate or do yoga exercises

A rested mind actually makes you feel more alive and energetic. Like the old saying less is more, a rested mind makes you more productive and less stressed out. I realize this sounds counterintuitive, but science backs it up.

Restorative Rest Under a Microscope

Dr. Herbert Benson, research scientist at the Harvard Medical School, calls restorative rest the relaxation response. He coined the phrase after studying Transcendental Meditation (TM) in practitioners who claimed they could lower their blood pressure with daily meditation. After distilling the basic techniques of TM, Benson's research shows that the relaxation response puts the brakes on the stress response. It lowers heart rate, blood pressure, and oxygen consumption, and reduces hypertension, arthritis, insomnia, depression, cancer, and anxiety.

Stress Vocab

The relaxation response, the opposite of the flight-or-flight response, is a physical state of deep rest that changes the physical and emotional responses to stress.

The Relaxation Response

The relaxation response is a great way to put the brakes on stress and calm your mind. You can practice this simple technique in just a few easy steps:

➤ Sit comfortably in a quiet place with your eyes closed.

➤ Start by deeply relaxing your muscles. Begin with the muscles of your feet working all the way up your body to your face.

➤ As you pay attention to your breathing, inhale through your nose and repeat a word or phrase that has special meaning to you while exhaling through your mouth. Dr. Benson suggests the word, *one* with each exhale as you breathe easily and naturally.

➤ When you notice your mind wandering (and it will), just passively bring your attention back to your breathing, repeating *one* as you exhale.

➤ Practice this technique for ten to twenty minutes a day for as many times a week as you can. It's better to open your eyes to keep track of time than use an alarm. Set aside a specific time and schedule your relaxation response sessions with the same commitment you would a professional meeting.

Recharging Your Batteries

Sit, stay, heal. Did you know that the calm you feel when you pet your goldendoodle, Siamese cat, or African gray parrot deactivates your stress response? Even watching fish swim in an aquarium can soothe you.

Pets keep you from getting lonely and depressed, keep you engaged, and make you feel cared about. Studies show that pets lower blood pressure and improve the survival rate for heart attack and stroke victims. The tactile stimulation from petting an animal releases endorphins and heightens the relaxation response. If it's not possible for you to own a pet, think about volunteering at an animal rescue center or visit a petting zoo or go horseback riding, where hands-on interactions are encouraged.

Internal Experiences for Resting Your Mind

Meaningful internal experiences quiet your mind and put it at rest. Here are just a few of the benefits you gain from creating a rested mind:

➤ Greater clarity of whether you are tense or rested

➤ Sharper concentration during tasks

➤ Lower reactivity to your usual stress triggers because your alarm system stays in the off mode as you walk around feeling more relaxed

➤ Quicker return to your relaxed state when you do get stressed-out

Contemplation, Spiritual Reflection, and Meditation

One of the best ways to quiet your mind is to set aside time for solitude and reflection. Studies show that spiritual practices such as prayer, meditation, and contemplation of nature neutralize stress hormones, putting the body at ease.

As a child growing up in the South, I remember church camp meetings, where believers fanned away sweltering heat as they worshipped under huge tents. I often peeked through slits in the tents to watch them raise their arms to the heavens, clap their hands, speak in tongues, run up and down aisles, and sometimes cut cartwheels in ecstasy as they became "slain in the spirit." Little did my boyhood eyes know they were engaging in religious practices that contributed to their stress resilience.

Recharging Your Batteries

Seekers who've had moments of deep spirituality say the main benefit is they don't feel alone. They feel a calm connection to a force bigger than themselves. They often speak of natural highs accompanying their experience. This state of euphoria occurs with the rush of a beautiful sunset, heightened bliss from deep meditation, relationship with a higher power in a 12-Step program, or spiritual connection through prayer.

Practitioners often describe these spiritual moments as oneness, being in the zone, runner's high, or creative flow—all of which are euphoric and, some would say, spiritual experiences. Not only do these practices leave you serene and rested, they boost your immune system and buffer stress.

Here are some of the scientific benefits of meaningful internal experiences:

➤ A view of nature from your hospital window can ease stress and contribute more to your recovery than certain drugs.

➤ People who go to church or meditate have a 35 percent reduced risk of death; plus they live longer and healthier lives than those who do not.

➤ Contemplative prayer, meditation, and yoga create calm and promote cognitive health, vitality, and long life.

➤ Optimists are more stress resistant and live longer and healthier lives than pessimists.

The takeaway is that there is not one spiritual prescription. Whether you're a nature lover, a regular at church or synagogue, a devotee to meditation, or a 12-Step follower, the important point is to find your own personal path that is meaningful, peaceful, and restorative. I devote full attention to mindfulness and meditation in the next two chapters.

Immerse Yourself in Deep Play

In her book, *Deep Play,* Diane Ackerman shows the importance of going deep into one pastime—instead of shallowly into three or four—that lets you sidestep reality. Deep play is a form of rapture created by an altered state that brings you restorative rest, joy, and well-being.

Stress Vocab

Deep Play is any activity that so engulfs you that you lose track of time and feel blanketed in its refuge, comforted from the stressors of daily life.

Jamey creates deep play by working with his orchids, which he describes as a type of meditation. He becomes so immersed that time stands still. There are no outside sounds, only the sounds of him digging, pulling, and raking. His awareness is so heightened that colors are more vivid and previously unnoticed objects stand out. That's what writing does for me. It picks me up and transports me to another zone where hours go by when it seems like only minutes have passed.

You, too, can create this state through an activity or pastime that you are passionate about, something you can become so immersed in that you lose all track of time. For some people, it's painting, sailing, gardening, playing tennis, dancing, singing, rock climbing, cooking, cycling, woodworking, skiing, or running. For others, it's wandering aimlessly in antique galleries, milling around attic sales, or browsing in bookstores.

Recharging Your Batteries

Think of a restorative activity that you enjoy, that helps you unwind. Recall the last time you did it. Was it a day, week, month, or year ago? Then think of something you've always wanted to do but never made time for. It can be something you're not good at, but that you'd like to explore. It doesn't have to culminate in a tangible product. It could even be something you deliberately do imperfectly. After you've thought of something you really like or think you'd like, dive into it. Whatever you choose, let it engulf you, take you away, lift your spirits, and rest your mind.

Emotions: When to Hold Them and When to Fold Them

In order to calm your mind, you can hold on to positive thoughts and feelings and let go of negative ones. It's important for you to hold on to the positive truth about yourself, even when it's hard to affirm it. At other times, it's essential to let go of built-up tension that keeps you stressed out. When you can hold positive thoughts and feelings and let go of negative ones, it brings tremendous stress relief. You can hold them with positive affirmations and fold them with cathartic release.

Positive Affirmations

Do you blush when someone praises you? Do you feel discomfort when you're applauded for a kind deed? Do you feel awkward when someone compliments you on how you look? If so, whether you're taking a test, making a speech, starting a new job, or struggling with parenting, making your own positive affirmations can help reduce stress.

Stress Vocab

Positive affirmations are positive present tense statements that reflect an emotional, mental, or physical state that you want to make your own.

Stop Going for the Jugular

Stress might dog you with negative self-doubt such as feeling like you can't do something before you even try. If this describes your state of mind, stop going for the jugular. Ask yourself what you'd say to your best friend or child if they thought they couldn't do something. You wouldn't say, "Of course you can't; you might as well give up." You would believe in them and encourage them with compassionate pep talks. You can give yourself that same compassionate encouragement.

Giving Yourself Positive Affirmations

When stress nips at your heels, try easing your mind with positive affirmations. These present tense statements are not tricks to convince you that a situation is better than it actually is. They are prescriptions of encouragement that you might not totally believe but you want to believe, and they are within your reach. Before you get into a situation, imagine the best of outcomes and tell yourself, "I can do what I set my mind to do, and I can do it well." Other examples of stress-reducing affirmations are:

➤ "My mind is calm and relaxed."

➤ "I manage stress with ease."

➤ "I feel emotionally well and serene."

Shock Absorber

As a reminder to yourself when you forget past validations, keep a computer file or bulletin board with affirming e-mails, letters, notes, gifts, and sayings that people send you. Look at them often to remember the truth about what others think of you. If someone praised you a week ago, that affirmation still stands even when stress trumps the good feelings. Put messages on your bathroom mirror, the back of a closet door, or your fridge, where you can see them each morning. Then hit your pause button now and then with a reminder of something positive about yourself.

Stress Vocab

Catharsis is the release of emotional tension by purging your thoughts and feelings through such modalities as writing, art, music, dance, or physical exercise.

Cathartic Release

Tired of your boss biting your head off? At the end of your rope with your neighbor's barking dog? Frustrated by a family member's constant complaining? If so, finding an outlet for your pent-up feelings might be in order.

One way to get this cathartic release is to vent by writing. Did you know that jotting down your thoughts, feelings, frustrations, and stressors can actually improve your health? Studies show that putting down your stressful experiences on computer or with pen and paper has positive physiological payoffs: enhanced immune system, reduction in severity of illness, and mental release of past troubling events.

Writing a Cathartic Letter

The purpose of writing a cathartic letter is for you to have a field day with your stress instead of keeping it bottled up. But this is a letter for your eyes only, not for the eyes of the person, place, or thing that stresses you out.

Start with "Dear (name of the person or situation)." Then start writing nonstop as fast as you can without lifting your pen off the paper or pausing your fingers on the keyboard. Forget everything your third grade teacher taught you about spelling, grammar, or handwriting. Try not to censor your feelings or edit your thoughts. Don't try to make sense of what you put down. Remember, this is a letter for you and no one else.

After you've finished, put the letter in a private place or destroy it. It has already served its purpose. You can repeat this exercise as many times as you need to. Once you have fully released your stressful feelings, make a list in your stress journal of the restorative qualities you'd like to replace them with (such as calmness, serenity, peace, joy). Then practice the relaxation response and picture in your mind's eye those qualities filling you up.

Questions still loom about the long-lasting benefits of catharsis. Some experts believe blowing off steam actually strengthens anger over time. But in the short term, this exercise can help you get out pent-up feelings, de-stress, and calm down. So blast away!

Mellow Out with Natural Alternative Calming Techniques

When you're stressed, your body stores the tension, making it tight and sore. To remedy this mind-body dilemma, Western culture has adopted certain Eastern practices. Among the most popular are hatha yoga, tai chi (pronounced tie-chee), and qigong (pronounced chee-gong). And gaining popularity in the United States is laughter yoga.

The common link shared by these ancient practices is the integration of mind, body, and spirit, and the emphasis on concentration of body movement, stretching, and controlled breathing. The outcome is a meditative feeling of calm, clear-mindedness, and well-being. When practiced regularly, these exercises can reduce cortisol levels, foster sleep, lower blood pressure, increase strength and flexibility, and enhance mental health. While laughter yoga, tai chi, and qigong are performed in a standing position, hatha yoga is usually practiced lying on a mat.

De-stressing IS a Laughing Matter

When was the last time you had a good belly laugh? Studies show that laughter yoga gives your body some of the same benefits as moderate physical exercise. You've probably always known that humor is good medicine, that you feel better within seconds after you laugh. That's because laughter reverses hormonal changes brought on by cortisol and activates the secretion of endorphins, the body's own painkiller.

Research shows that laughing—even fake laughing—for just one minute a day dampens stress, eases pain, lowers blood pressure, stokes your immune system, and brightens your mental outlook. Capitalizing on these benefits, laughter yoga is built around forced laughter until it feels real. The science of laughter yoga is that even if you start with pretend laughing, your body can't tell the difference, and momentarily the laughter erases all your worries and relieves your mind of stress.

Recharging Your Batteries

Laughter yoga is a free-form enterprise and simple to do. It helps when you do this exercise with another person because laughter is contagious. Here's how:

➤ In a standing position, look upward and hold your arms wide apart above your head.

➤ Start with forced laughing, engaging your shoulders, arms, face, and belly until the laughter starts to feel real.

➤ Continue for as long as you can, letting it rip: *Ahhh-hahaha-whoohoohoo-ha-heeheehee!*

➤ After a few minutes of hearty belly laughing, see if you don't notice an instant lift from the exercise.

Next time you can't get to the gym, try "laughter-cise": *Ha ha ha-Ho ho ho-He he he!*

Hatha Yoga

The ancient practice of hatha yoga is the most common type of yoga and the best for starters. The pace is slow and steady, and the poses are easier than those of some other types of yoga. Hatha yoga blends several surefire basics that work directly on your stress response:

➤ Stretching

➤ Body poses

➤ Controlled breathing

➤ Focused attention

➤ Mental awareness

➤ The meditative process

The basic technique is to stretch and concentrate on holding different postures as you control your breathing. Yoga draws you away from ruminating thoughts and worries as you move through poses with names like the cobra or the mountain that require balance and concentration. Staying focused on your body and breath gives your linear brain a long-overdue break. After just one session, you can come away with a quieter mind, feeling lighter, refreshed, and clearheaded.

Benefits of Practicing Yoga

When practiced consistently, research bears out that yoga brings down your cortisol level and fosters sleep. Studies show that you get a 65 percent increase in dopamine squirts with certain types of yoga. Plus, the practice lowers blood pressure, improves blood flow, boosts cognitive functioning, combats fatigue, and raises a sense of well-being. Breathing and stretching forms of yoga can increase gamma-aminobutyric acid (GABA) levels in your brain by as much as 27 percent. GABA is associated with reduced depression and anxiety.

Stress Vocab

Hatha yoga is a stress-reduction technique that includes controlled breath concentration while gently stretching the body and forming different poses in a series of slow, steady movements.

In one study, stressed-out caregivers of patients with dementia showed an improvement in physical and emotional functioning after doing yoga. In another study, Army veterans suffering from post-traumatic stress disorder drastically reduced their stress level after practicing yoga twice a week for ten weeks. So if yoga is effective at calming such extreme stress, imagine what it can do for stress caused by dealing with the daily grind.

I can personally attest to yoga's effectiveness. The yoga classes I've taken have left me with a deep sense of calm, clarity, relaxation, and well-being. Attending a yoga class where you can nail down the basics is the best way to learn the correct poses and prevent injury. If you have physical limitations, trained instructors will encourage you not to exceed them and to move at your own pace and comfort level. You can find yoga classes just about anywhere—the gym, college campuses, hospitals, senior centers, and trendy health studios.

Stress Vocab

Qigong is a meditative practice that balances and increases your vital life energy flow through body movement, creating less stressful and healthier mind, body, and spirit.

Tai Chi and Qigong

Every morning when I awoke in China, I was blown away by the sight of groups of people—young and old—moving in graceful, slow-motion synchrony in parks, university campuses, and city centers. That morning ritual called qigong, common in many parts of Asia, has gained popularity in the United States, along with tai chi, as a method of unwinding from a hectic lifestyle.

Stress Vocab

Tai chi, originally designed for self-defense, is a self-paced series of slow, flowing body movements that require concentration and lead to the relaxation of body and mind.

Tai chi is another great way to reduce stress and mellow out while you condition your body. Standing, you move constantly, slowly, and harmoniously, stretching in a seamless flow from one posture to the next. As with yoga, tai chi holds your attention in the present as you concentrate on breathing, stretching, and a series of prescribed body movements. One study found that tai chi boosts immunity and resistance to the shingles virus in older adults.

I practice qigong. Although the movements are similar to tai chi, qigong is an "internal" martial art with movements that are simpler, easier to learn, and less sweeping. But like tai chi, qigong is an ancient Chinese practice of slow, graceful movements, visualization, and breathing. Qigong allows you to connect with your body and become more aware of your life force energy. This energy balance creates lasting calming and health benefits for mind and body that continue long after practice sessions.

Both tai chi and qigong take time to learn the different body positions. The best way is to take a class and learn from an experienced instructor. Once you've got the poses down pat, your body will remember each pose as you move rhythmically and gently through the series. The outcome of letting your body do the "thinking" puts you in a peaceful and invigorated state.

The good news is that tai chi and qigong are safe and easy for anyone of any age. It is especially suitable for senior citizens and other people who are prohibited from vigorous exercise. They can actually help people with Parkinson's disease and other illnesses. If you're not sure these movements are right for you, discuss it with your family doctor first.

Herbal Supplements

Some natural herbs are said to relax the mind and body. Although the effectiveness of natural supplements is inconclusive, many people champion their use.

You can find several natural remedies that are said to have mild mitigating effects on stress at natural health food stores. Here are a few of the remedies:

➤ Melatonin regulates your sleep rhythms

➤ Valerian helps with insomnia and stress

➤ GABA induces sleep

➤ Saint John's wort is considered a mild antidepressant

➤ Amino acids such as L-Tryptophan (found in warm milk, cheese, and poultry) and 5-HTP act as calming supplements, sleep aids, and antidepressants.

Truth Serum

The scientific evidence on the effectiveness of herbal supplements in easing stress is still inconclusive. In one study, patients with generalized anxiety took chamomile extract, a calming remedy. After eight weeks, the chamomile reduced anxiety and worries much like prescribed antidepressants do. But a lot more research needs to be done before I can give herbal supplements a hardy two thumbs up as a bona fide stress reliever.

Most of these supplements are sold over the counter, except for L-Tryptophan, which was taken off the market in the United States. But before taking supplements, be sure to check with your physician, especially if you're taking other prescription drugs. Although called natural, herbal remedies are still medicines that affect your body and mind. And when taken with prescriptions, the interaction could have adverse effects.

Bend with Life's Curveballs

Tropical palms are stress resistant, not because they stand rigid and hard against tropical storms, but because they bend with the wind. Bending (fully accepting) with life's stressors, instead of fighting them, can help you score big, too. Of course, that's a hard concept to grasp, in the heat of a stressful moment. But going ballistic won't keep the game from getting rained out, get you out of a traffic jam, or keep your plane from delay. Once you bend with a difficult condition beyond your control, you can let it go and reduce your stress level. When you acknowledge the things you can't control, accept them, and turn your attention to the things you can control, it brings calm. In a calm state of mind, you can figure out a strategy to manage the stressor.

The Doctor Of Calm Is In

If a man has nothing to eat, fasting is the most intelligent thing he can do

—Hermann Hesse

Surrendering to conditions beyond your control doesn't remove all the stress, but it reduces a lot of it. My prescription: Ask yourself if you're resisting an unwanted life stressor beyond your control. Bending once daily to a stressor is the recommended starting dose to provide sustained serenity over twenty-four hours. This once-daily dosing may be used alone or in combination with other stress-reduction techniques discussed in this chapter. Here's to outsmarting your stress!

CHAPTER 12

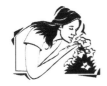 # Mindful Awareness and Stress Reduction

---

In This Chapter

➤ What mindful awareness is

➤ How mindfulness techniques reduce stress

➤ Your mindfulness score

➤ Practicing mindful awareness

In this chapter, you'll learn about mindful awareness along with different levels of mindfulness practices. You'll get an idea of your mindful score and how to hone your skills using mindfulness techniques to relieve stress. You'll find some simple exercises to practice that will help you become more mindful in your everyday activities.

Are You on Autopilot or Are You Awake at the Wheel?

Many years ago, I was in a New York City cab on the way to appear on a television show. I remember telling my traveling companion, "I want to hurry up and get to the hotel so I can relax." When I think back, I wonder why I couldn't relax right then and there. Why wait? If you start to watch, you too will be amazed by how your mind constantly tries to figure out how to maximize pleasure and minimize pain.

Are you in fast-forward much of the time, trying to get to the good stuff—the nirvana of pleasure—missing out on what's happening now? You know what I mean. You have to get through the traffic jam instead of *being* in the traffic jam. You have to hop in and out of the shower to get to work instead of *being* in the shower. You have to hurry up with dinner so you can watch TV instead of *being* present with dinner preparation.

Recharging Your Batteries

When you lose your attunement, you forfeit yourself to a mind fog that engulfs you, steeping you in its own stress juices. I call these brownouts—the side effects of tuning out the here and now; memory loss of conversations or momentary forgetfulness because you're "out of your present mind." But your presence of mind gives you the power to flip the pattern around, landing you in the driver's seat, putting you back in charge. When you wake up and fully engage in each moment, you rediscover your daily world in a completely different way. And your life takes on a fresh glow.

How many people do you notice in a day (yourself included) driving while texting, or strolling in the park on a beautiful day, cell phone glued to an ear, or eating lunch, typing a memo, and talking on the phone simultaneously? We have become a nation immune to the present moment.

Is your mind busy with so many thoughts coming and going that you don't have a chance to pause and catch your breath? Do you frantically work on projects, focused on the next item on the agenda, worrying if the boss will like the finished product, or thinking about what you'll be doing this weekend? These out-of-the-moment episodes create loads of stress and disconnect you from yourself and your surroundings. Before you know it, you're mired in your own stress soup.

Your Wandering Mind

It's human nature for your mind to wander from time to time. In fact, it could be wandering right now. You could be thinking about what you ate for lunch and what you "should" have eaten. You could be worried about unpaid bills or about an unfinished project, ruminating about how you'll meet the deadline. Or you might be replaying in your head an argument you had with your spouse.

When your mind wanders too much, it could be stressing you out or at the very least preventing you from fully relaxing. Your wandering mind misses the beautiful sunset and the warm breeze brushing against your face or the soft music on your car radio, or the chance of having a meaningful moment with the person next to you.

Truth Serum

Harvard researchers found that the human mind wanders 47 percent of the time and that when you stray, you pay. They contacted 2,200 people around the world at random over several days and asked them each to use their iPhone to report what they were doing, thinking about, and feeling. Nearly half of the world's population was mentally absent during such activities as personal grooming, commuting, cooking, working, taking a walk, shopping, and so on.

The Harvard study concluded that when your mind wanders, you're more stressed out and unhappy than when you stay in the here and now. No matter what people were doing, even if they were working overtime, vacuuming the house, or sitting in traffic, they were happier if they were focused on the activity instead of thinking about something else.

Scientists say the way you use your mind can determine how much stress you have. Keeping your focus in the present instead of ruminating about what already happened (which you can't change anyway) or about what might happen (which you can't control anyway) keeps your stress level down and makes for a happier life.

What is Mindfulness?

There's a way to reclaim your life: through mindfulness—the ability to pay compassionate, nonjudgmental attention to what you're thinking and feeling, and to what's happening around you in the present moment.

Stress Vocab

Mindfulness is the practice of paying attention to your everyday life experiences from moment to moment, being aware of what you're experiencing while you're experiencing it, and accepting without judgment whatever arises whether it is a thought, feeling, or body sensation.

Sidestepping the Mind Fogs

You can neutralize stress with mindfulness practices by taking four actions:

> ➤ Keep your focus in the present moment

> ➤ Move at a steady, calm pace

> ➤ Be attuned to yourself and your surroundings

> ➤ Accept without judgment whatever arises in each moment

This practice isn't as easy as it sounds. Even though you may not be aware of it, you're probably judging yourself and your experience of others much of the time. Think about the last time you took a shower or brushed your teeth (I hope it wasn't too long ago). Chances are that you were thinking about other things in your life besides what you were doing at that moment. And your mind might have been miles away from your body, caught up in thought streams about future or past judgments.

Shock Absorber

Take time right now to notice your thoughts. In a relaxed position, put yourself fully into the present moment. Try watching the thoughts streaming through your mind with a nonjudgmental attitude. You don't have to do anything but pay attention to them. Don't try to change or fix them. Just be aware of them. Are the thoughts centered on the future or the past; or are they focused in the present? Are they calm and serene or worried and anxious? You'll probably notice that they're preparing you to react to situations with more stress than necessary. Or they might be replaying a negative situation that you could've handled differently. This type of paying attention to your mind is called mindful awareness.

Stress-Reduction Benefits of Mindfulness

Experts say that mindfulness techniques are powerful stress antidotes. Studies show that the way you pay attention in the present moment directly affects your body and brain, your feelings and thoughts, and your interpersonal relationships. Mindful techniques harness the social circuitry of the brain, enabling you to be attuned to your own mind.

And there's lots of proof. Scientists report that practicing mindfulness slows down your heart rate and brain wave patterns and boosts your immune system and cardiac functioning. With regular meditation, you have less stress, fewer health problems, improved relationships, and a longer life. Studies show that mindfulness techniques help you work with difficult feelings and develop a sense of well-being.

Truth Serum

A body of research from the University of Massachusetts Medical School shows that mindfulness meditation improves your ability to act instead of react under stress. Regular practice activates your parasympathetic nervous system and equips you to face stress without getting frazzled. Wake Forest University researchers found that brain function improves after just four days of mindfulness meditation. In that study, meditators showed significant gains in working memory, verbal fluency, and executive function. And stressed-out people who underwent a mindfulness training program at West Virginia University reduced their stress by 54 percent and their medical symptoms by 46 percent.

Where Do You Fall on the Mindfulness Scale?

You can think of mindfulness on one end of a scale and mindlessness on the other end. Studies show that mindlessness leads to stress-related mental and physical problems. But mindfulness promotes stress-resistant qualities. Take a look at the vast difference and see where you fall on the scale:

➤ Mindfulness: Present-moment awareness
  Mindlessness: Future or past oriented

➤ Mindfulness: Self-compassion
  Mindlessness: Self-judgment

➤ Mindfulness: Self-care
  Mindlessness: Self-neglect

➤ Mindfulness: Calmness and serenity
  Mindlessness: Worry and anxiety

➤ Mindfulness: Rest and digest response (PNS activation)
  Mindlessness: Stress response (SNS activation)

➤ Mindfulness: Self-attuned, or awake
  Mindlessness: Autopilot, or asleep

➤ Mindfulness: Balance
Mindlessness: Imbalance

➤ Mindfulness: Security
Mindlessness: Insecurity

When you compare the extremes, it's clear that mindless living creates greater stress. It distracts you from paying attention to your greatest asset: your mind.

Shock Absorber

Take time right now to try your hand at this simple exercise:

➤ Turn your attention to your fingers and focus there for a minute.

➤ Wiggle your fingers and notice how this sensory experience feels. Focus on how the wiggling looks and sounds. Do you hear any crackling in your joints or sounds of skin against skin? What else are you aware of?

➤ Notice if you judge yourself or the exercise, or if you have trouble staying focused.

➤ After you've finished, jot down your thoughts in your stress journal.

Did this simple exercise give you an immediate connection to the present moment, or did your judgment interfere with you being fully engaged? If you were fully engaged during the exercise, you might've noticed that previous worries or stressful thoughts were absent. Write in your stress journal what this experience was like for you.

Did you fall on the scale at one end or somewhere in between? To get a clearer picture of where you fall, you can compute your mindful score by taking the test in Appendix A called Are You a Mindful Marvel or a Mindless Menace?

Creating Mindful Conditions

Whatever your score, don't despair. The remainder of this chapter gives you the tools you need to awaken to a place of mindful acceptance. Chances are that you might get so used to living with stress and chaos that it becomes a habit. You might even catch yourself adding stress to your busy life, even when you don't mean to. For that reason, it's important to intentionally create mindful conditions in your life.

Steps to Slow Down Your Pace

Ask yourself how often you race through the day without pausing to consider who you really are and what you want out of life. Creating mindful conditions for yourself is the starting point. Consider some of the following steps to slow your pace and bring gentle awareness to your thoughts and feelings:

➤ Set aside times to eat slower instead of eating with what one mindfulness expert called "the three g's," gobble, gulp, and go.

➤ Avoid eating and working while standing, walking, driving, or on the run.

➤ Slow down by driving and walking slower and saying no when you already have commitments.

➤ Give yourself time cushions when setting important deadlines.

➤ Do just one activity at a time, bringing all of your conscious attention to it.

➤ Delegate and prioritize tasks if you can, and eliminate those that are the least important or unnecessary.

➤ Schedule extra driving time to destinations and stretch time between appointments so you're not rushed.

Trending Now from the Smart Files

Many health benefits result from practicing mindfulness. Here are a few:

➤ Researchers at the University of Rochester Medical Center found that primary care physicians who practiced mindfulness increased their stress resilience and reduced burnout and mood disturbance.

➤ Swiss scientists reported that multiple sclerosis patients who completed eight weeks of mindfulness training were less fatigued and depressed, and their quality of life was improved.

➤ In Sweden, patients with irritable bowel syndrome who took mindfulness training had a 42 percent decrease in frequency and severity of overall pain, bloating, and flatulence, compared to patients without the training.

➤ In Canada, patients with breast and prostate cancer who underwent eight weeks of mindfulness training, showed a decrease in stress symptoms and an increase in quality of life.

Having a Mindful Awareness Moment

You've probably heard the saying "Life is what happens while you're doing other things." Mindful awareness plucks you out of "mind stupors" and plops you smack dab into what's happening in the moment. It opens you up to the deep mystery of being alive without the need for numbing yourself with future worries, frenzied activities, or multitasking. You might even begin to notice a fascination with the simple things, beauty in the ordinary, richness in the humdrum.

Easing Yourself into the Present

Cultivating mindfulness in your life takes willingness, awareness, and a shift in your perspective. Here's a real-life example to show you what I mean:

When it came to his high-pressured job, Jason squeezed every second out of his personal life. Most nights he came home beat, his two excited boys jumping all over him. As a way to reduce his stress, Jason decided to ask his wife and kids to give him fifteen minutes to unwind when he came home from work. But after learning about mindfulness, Jason had a lightbulb moment. He realized that the sweetest times in his life were when his sons tackled him at the front door. Why would he push away those tender moments, knowing that he wouldn't get a do-over someday?

So instead of putting off his most treasured moments, Jason put himself into them and savored each second. The shift actually relaxed and rejuvenated him more than a fifteen-minute reprieve. Instead of changing his outer world, Jason's revelation enabled him to switch his inner world. This is the first step in mindful awareness: close attention to what's right before your eyes instead of rushing past it, pushing it away, or trying to change it.

Levels of Mindfulness Practices

As with any new activity, you can practice mindfulness at different levels. You can weave formal and informal practices into your life, depending on your schedule and how far you want to go with it. This chapter is concerned mainly with informal level 1 practices— mindful awareness as you go through your daily activities, which is a good entry into a mindfulness experience if this is new territory for you.

Practicing mindfulness is like a physical fitness program; you start slowly and build up your concentration and strength of presence. If you're out of shape and want to get physically fit, you start out small by doing things like taking the stairs instead of the elevator, parking a distance from the mall instead of parking near the entrance. In the same way, you start your entry into mindfulness with practices that are already built into your day. Without changing your routines, you can make small attitude adjustments in your daily activities like eating, cooking, walking, and working.

Level 1: Open Awareness Practice

Level 1 mindfulness is peacefully observing your awareness of everything you do. It can be any brief activity that makes you awake and aware of what's happening as it happens in the flow of your daily routines. You can intentionally walk with present-moment awareness by bringing your attention to the sensations of your feet against the ground, or noting the feel of the open sky, sights, and sounds around you as you make your way to the parking garage.

Recharging Your Batteries

When you weed in the garden, you can pay attention to the plants' resistance against your hands as you tug, and the sound of stubborn roots and smell of fresh soil as you unearth the weeds from their home. When you clean the toilet bowl, brush your teeth, drive your car, or cook a pot of soup, you can step out of your thought stream and make yourself fully present in the activity. While waiting in the doctor's office, you could practice mindful listening. In line at the grocery store, you could tune in to your body sensations. Stuck in traffic, you could practice mindful breathing.

You can even practice open awareness right now. As you read on, you might find your mind wandering from time to time. Just be aware of your wandering mind, let it be okay, and gently bring it back to the words on the printed page.

Level 2: Focused Attention Practice

If you have the time and interest, you can take your mindfulness practice to the next level. Level 2 practice is a more formal schedule that involves dedicated times to focused attention. The equivalent in building your exercise regimen would be working out on your StairMaster for twenty minutes a day or going to the gym for an aerobics class three times a week. Typically, in level 2 mindfulness, you set aside time in the day to sit down in a quiet place. You focus your attention on your breathing, a mantra, or an object of concentration.

Level 3: Intensive Event Practice

If you want to go hog wild, you can attend an intensive event at a mindfulness workshop or retreat center. Mindfulness intensives are held in a specific place with a group of people, often in silence, for an extended period of time. The exercise equivalent would be biking in the Tuscan countryside for a week or going to a weight-loss spa for several days. There are many excellent retreat centers across the United States. The major ones are listed in Appendix B.

Practicing Mindfulness Exercises

Informal mindfulness exercises can reduce the stress that accumulates during your daily activities, generating more energy to carry you through demanding situations. Paying closer attention to the routines that you usually fast-forward through will give you fresh, new insights to your life. If your mind kicks into high gear and tries to hurry you through these exercises, take a deep breath and gently bring your attention back to the present moment and the task at hand. Studies show that because this slowing down changes your body chemistry, you'll be more peaceful on the inside and more productive in the long run.

Take a Mindful Morning Shower

Try a mindful exercise during your morning shower. Pay attention to the sounds and feel of thousands of beads of water splashing against your skin. Hear the rushing water beating against your shower curtain and smacking against the tub. As you lather your body, be aware of the smell and feel of the slippery soap gliding over your skin, the soap bubbles swelling and popping on your neck, arms, and chest. Notice how the water feels rolling down your body, the fresh fragrance of shampoo and its cleansing feel against your scalp. As you dry off, feel the fabric of the towel against your skin. Continue your present-moment awareness while brushing your teeth and going through the rest of your morning routine.

Prepare a Mindful Meal

Prepare a meal as if you're cooking it for the first time. Pay close attention as you assemble the ingredients. Notice the unique character of each vegetable, fruit, or piece of meat—the myriad of colors, diverse smells, and varied textures of foods. Even the sounds are different as you chop, slice, cut, grind, and pound. You might pop an ingredient into your mouth, noting its texture against your tongue and its unique taste. As you combine the different ingredients, notice the visual transformation as they become one. While you're cooking, observe the chemical process as the separate items morph into a collected whole. Inhale the aroma, noting if you can still identify the unique smells of each ingredient or simply one succulent blend. When you sit to eat, take in the smells and colors of the meal before you dig in.

Wake Up! Are You Out of Your Present Mind?

After you've completed a few of these exercises, you might discover another world that you hadn't noticed before. Ask yourself the following questions and record your thoughts and feelings in your stress journal:

➤ As you looked at your usual routines in a new way, what did you notice?

➤ Were you aware that there's more happening around you and inside you than you realized?

➤ Did your thoughts kick into gear and try to rush you through the activity?

➤ Were your old stressors along for the ride or did they stay behind?

➤ As you notice where your mind is from moment to moment, do you feel more connected to yourself? Does your life seem more vivid?

The Doctor Of Calm Is In

Much of the time we're going through life, inattentive to what's happening, trying to get to the Shangri-la of pleasure, missing out on what's happening, here and now.

—Ronald Siegel

Do you get lost in past thoughts or future concerns instead of being present? These out-of-the-moment episodes are roadblocks to relaxation. They disconnect you from yourself and your surroundings and keep your stress response activated. My prescription: Watch your mind, noticing where it goes from moment to moment, for the next twenty-four hours. Note the difference between when you are present and when your mind drifts to the past or future. When you find your mind wandering—even if it's now as you read these words—gently bring it back to the present. Continue to notice where your mind is in each moment until tension subsides and you feel more relaxed. Here's to outsmarting your stress!

CHAPTER 13

 # Meditation Practices and Stress Resilience

In This Chapter

➤ What meditation is

➤ Benefits of meditation for relieving stress

➤ Types of meditation

➤ How meditation helps with judgment and distress

In this chapter, you'll learn about formal meditation, as well as the main types of meditation. You'll learn the basic steps of formal meditation, what you need to meditate, and how to get started. And you'll find examples of guided meditations, get to try one on for size, and see how to create your own. Plus, you'll learn how to observe your thoughts that cause stress and how to stay calm during unpleasant emotional states.

What is Meditation?

Nowadays there's a lot to keep you up at night. Stress might have you doing a lot of hand-wringing. Your attention might be pulled in a million directions at once, or you might feel like someone has taken a nine iron to your head. Whatever your distress, meditation offers practical tools for stress relief.

In previous chapters, you had a chance to try your hand at informal types of meditation. So you might have already enjoyed the benefits of sitting quietly and meditative breathing, as well as dealing with stray thoughts and your wandering mind. This chapter builds on those skills, blending them together and taking you deeper into more formal meditation, where you focus your attention.

Stress Vocab

Meditation is the practice of quieting your mind by directing your attention to a focal point such as your breath, an image, or a sound.

Although formal meditation practices have been around for thousands of years in the Far East, they got a bum rap when first introduced in this country in the 1970s. Many cynics scoffed at the idea of fringe mystical practices involving gurus, weird chants, shoulder-length hair, burning incense, and, in some cases, drugged-out hippies looking for another way to zone out. Meditation was clearly misunderstood. But not anymore.

Ten Million Americans Plus Hard Science Can't Be Wrong

Today, about 10 million Americans practice some form of meditation. And hard science has shown that meditation is a highly effective technique for reducing stress. As a result of these eye-popping findings, people are buzzing about meditation as one of the most beneficial stress-reduction tools available today. Some airports even house meditation rooms for passengers plodding through terminals at all hours of the day and night.

Truth Serum

It's no longer a question whether meditation changes your brain. Through the advancement of neuroimaging techniques, studies show that there are structural differences between the brains of meditators and those who don't meditate. Scientists know without a doubt that long-term stress impairs thinking, focused attention, and executive functioning.

On the flip side, brain scans show that people who meditate regularly have an increase of gray matter density and less brain shrinkage and overall cognitive decline. One study of patients with recurrent mood disorders reported that meditation prevented relapses of depression. In another study, researchers reported that when meditators heard sounds of people suffering, they had stronger activation levels in the empathy parts of their brain than non-meditators. Who wouldn't want their empathetic spouses or partners to take out the trash or clean the kitchen because they know you like it?

Benefits of Meditation

Hard evidence reveals that meditation has the following benefits:

➤ Puts the brakes on your stress response and activates your calming response

➤ Sharpens your alertness, ability to focus, attention span, and awareness of your surroundings

➤ Strengthens your emotional stability, and reduces reactions under stress, anxiety, and depression

➤ Increases your ability to empathize and be compassionate

➤ Enhances your physical health, lowers blood pressure, improves memory, strengthens your immune system, and increases the gray matter in your brain

➤ Provides you with a renewed outlook, pleasant feelings, and deeper appreciation for life

It's Easier than You Think

So with benefits like these who wouldn't want to meditate, right? Not so fast. If you haven't meditated before, you might be thinking what a lot of people think, that meditation is another complicated tool that you don't have time for. But as you read on, you'll realize that meditating isn't as complicated as it's made out to be. In fact, you'll see that the advantages of meditating far outweigh the disadvantages.

The Goal of Meditation: Not to Have a Goal

The goal of meditation is not to zone out, withdraw from life, or get rid of unpleasant thoughts. It's not a religious practice, nor does it require you to change your beliefs or commit to a particular religious doctrine. Meditation is a tool to help you investigate the habitual workings of your mind, how your thoughts routinely create stress, and how you can get them to relax. The goal of meditation is not to have a goal other than to recognize your pattern of latching on to negative, judgmental thoughts about your daily life: right and wrong, for and against, yes and no, needing things to be one way or another instead of accepting everything just as it is in the present.

By simply noticing your thoughts, you start to see how many thoughts are worries about the future or regrets about the past. As you recognize your thoughts are just thoughts, not truths, you learn not to make too much of them. It is this recognition that melts your stress away.

Types of Meditation

There are many types of meditation. But most can be put into two main categories: insight meditation (mindful open awareness), discussed in the previous chapter, and focused-attention meditation (concentration), the focus of this chapter.

Insight Meditation

Mindfulness, or open awareness practice, which I discussed in the previous chapter, is a form of insight meditation. With insight meditation, you bring your full attention (your vision, hearing, touch, smell, and taste) to your body and mind in present time without attempting to change anything. The goal is simply to observe what is happening within and around you without judgment.

Insight meditation gives you an objective awareness (or insight) of situations or events causing you stress, and helps you pinpoint avenues for greater stress resilience.

From my own practice of insight meditation, I can attest to what many practitioners say: it gives me an outsider's view of how I'm living my life. It helps me sort through my perspective about my life and review the feelings I have about it. It provides many aha moments, or insights that help me make changes in response to hard-hitting stressors.

Stress Vocab

Mantra—which literally means "a tool of thought"—is a special image, word, or sound that is used in meditation as a point of focus such as *one, om, calm,* or *peace.*

Focused-Attention Meditation

This chapter is concerned with focused attention in which you concentrate on an object of meditation. You focus on your breath, a word, or a mantra. A good example of focused attention is the relaxation response (described in Chapter 11). You'll remember that I described the basic steps that Herbert Benson distilled from Transcendental Meditation in which you concentrate on your breath and a word that has special meaning to you. As you focus on a word, sound, or object, the practice takes you away from thinking about your job being on the chopping block, bills piling up, or a relationship going down the toilet. It activates other areas of your brain that calm you and leave you with a steady mind-set to face life's inevitable ups and downs. Your concentration brings your mind to the here and now instead of letting it drift.

One specific type of focused-attention meditation is compassion meditation in which you concentrate on a compassionate thought or image that is designed to enhance your ability to empathize with the suffering of others. In compassion meditation, you pay attention to your emotions toward others and recognize your common humanity. This type of meditation helps relieve stress and softens your responses to stress.

Shock Absorber

There are many myths that can keep you from taking even the first step toward formal meditation. But truth be told, you don't need to assemble elaborate equipment, burn incense, twist yourself into a pretzel cross-legged on the floor, play weird music, clear your mind of all thoughts, or sit for hours. All you need to start is five or ten minutes, a comfortable chair or cushion, and a place where you won't be interrupted or distracted. Find a quiet spot in your home, office, or garden, devoid of blasting TV, blinking computer screen, intrusive cell phone pings, or frenzied pets and children. Sit upright with your spine straight in a chair or on the floor. And you're ready to roll.

How to Practice Meditating

One of the simplest and easiest forms of focused-attention meditation is to use your breath as a focal point. The actual practice of this meditation is realizing your attention has strayed and bringing your mind back to your breath, linking your mind and body together in the present moment. Once you do this over and over again, your meditation practice helps you stay more in the here and now as you move through your daily routines.

Basic Steps for Beginning Meditation

I recommend that you meditate for only five or ten minutes to start, gradually increasing your sit time to twenty or thirty minutes once or twice a day over time.

Once you find a comfortable, quiet place to meditate, begin to relax your body. You can close your eyes, or leave them open or half-open. Then, you're ready to practice this simple technique by following these basic steps:

➤ Start to pay attention to your breathing, noticing the air moving in through your nose and out through your mouth. Allow your breath to move naturally as you observe it.

➤ Breathe in and out as you connect with each inhalation and exhalation, noticing how it feels as you begin the inhalation, how it feels as you are between the inhalation and the exhalation and the sensations of your breath on the exhalation.

➤ Follow your breath through to a full cycle from the beginning of an inhalation, where your lungs are relatively full, back to where they're empty.

➤ Notice the rise and fall of your belly; the air moving in and out of your nostrils.

➤ As thoughts and feelings arise in the form of judgments—wondering if you're doing this right, thinking about what you have to do later, questioning if it's worth your time to be doing this—simply observe them without added judgment and let them go.

➤ Once you realize your thoughts have hijacked your attention, gently bring your attention back and focus on your breath.

➤ Each time you notice your attention leaving your breath, bring your awareness back to concentrating on your breathing.

➤ If your mind gets caught in a chain of thought, gently step out of the thought stream and come back to the sensations of your breath. Each time it wanders off, continue bringing it back again for the amount of time you have designated to practice.

➤ Notice any body discomfort, hunger pangs, sensations of hot or cold, an itch, but don't do anything about them; just breathe and watch. Remind yourself there's nowhere else to be, nothing else to do but notice your breath in this moment. All you're doing is training your mind to be present right now.

➤ After the designated amount of time, gently open your eyes and bring your attention back into the room, taking in the colors and textures around you. Stretch and breathe normally, noticing how much more vivid and acute your awareness is and how much more connected you feel to yourself and the moment.

Recharging Your Batteries

If your mind is still after meditating, if you feel relaxed and rested, and if you have a calmer approach to stress, chances are you're meditating correctly. In the long term, you know meditation is working because you're less reactive to upsetting events, you worry less, you're more grounded in the here and now instead of the past or future, you're more adaptable and stress resilient, and you have a deeper appreciation for life. In other words, your batteries feel recharged most of the time.

Studies show that intense forms of meditation such as Transcendental Meditation and other forms of focused-attention meditation raise serotonin levels in your blood, creating heightened visual imagery and enhanced sensory experiences.

Cultivating a Daily Practice that Works for You

If you practice some form of meditation on a regular basis, it can bring you tremendous stress relief and elevate your mood. When you get the hang of it, you can practice once or twice daily or several times a week. Here are some tips to get you started on a meditation routine that works for you:

> ➤ Decide on a time and day that you can fully devote to sitting for a period of time without rushing to another pressure or deadline.

> ➤ Stick to the same days and times as much as you can. It doesn't matter whether it's morning, afternoon, or evening. What matters is that you have a consistent routine.

> ➤ Designate a specific place and go there each time you meditate. You can use a quiet corner or any spot free of distractions.

> ➤ Consider furnishing your spot with special reminders that draw you in, such as a photograph of a nature scene, image of an inspirational spiritual person, smell of a candle.

> ➤ Start with five minutes. Then commit to sitting for fifteen to twenty minutes as you become more comfortable with your routine. Make sure you're comfortable in your upright sitting posture (spine straight), whether in a chair or on a meditation cushion.

> ➤ Remind yourself that the point of meditation is not to have a goal other than to observe your breath and your thoughts, feelings, and physical sensations without judging them as a particular good or bad experience. Let it be whatever it is.

> ➤ Consider joining a meditation group. Joining a group does not commit you to becoming a follower of any particular discipline. But many practitioners say that having a meditation group heightens the experience and supports the commitment to the practice. You can also check out Appendix B for meditation resources for beginners.

Shock Absorber

Are you wondering where you can find a stress reduction meditation class? Meditation classes are conducted around the country in churches and synagogues, community centers, and hospitals. Medical centers at Duke University, the Mayo Clinic, Yale University, and Massachusetts General Hospital offer mindfulness-based stress reduction (MBSR) workshops, inspired by the pioneering work of Jon Kabat-Zinn. And many counselors run meditation groups for clients using the MBSR model. Plus, retreat centers in various regions of the country offer week-long meditation and yoga classes for beginners and advanced students. Check out Appendix B for some of these destinations.

Meditating with Guided Imagery

After a demanding day of feeling overwhelmed, visualizations are a great resource to shut down your stress response and ease your mind and body into a state of relaxation. Visualizations allow you to conjure up serene images and scenes in your mind and focus on them. As you create calming images, your body automatically responds by calming down, melting away your stress.

Stress Vocab

Guided meditations refer to the step-by-step instruction on using the power of your imagination to evoke calm, relaxing mind and body responses.

The intentional use of visualizations can elevate your mood, reduce worry and stress, improve success motivation, and raise athletic performance. They can even enhance your immune system and aid in many types of diseases.

Guided Visualizations

Guided visualizations are scripted, usually directed by an audio recording or the written word. You are guided to a peaceful scene and instructed to bring up images of a particular theme.

Here's how it works:

➤ Get comfortable in a relaxed position in a quiet place where you can put yourself fully into this journey.

➤ Focus on your breathing. Take a few deep breaths in through your nose and out through your mouth. Get connected with your breathing.

➤ Let go of thoughts about what happened earlier today. And forget about what you have to do later today or tomorrow. Let this be a time just for you. Continue to be aware of your breathing and relax.

➤ Imagine yourself in a place or in a previous memory where you feel comfort, joy, relaxation, or gratitude. Common images are soft, puffy clouds, a green meadow, the seashore, a bubbling mountain brook, or being in the company of a pet, child, or loved one.

➤ As you are guided, imagine being with the person, place, or thing, putting yourself fully there by using your five senses to vividly experience what it looks, sounds, smells, tastes, and feels like to your touch.

As another example, try this one on for size:

➤ Imagine yourself lying under a large shade tree in a meadow blanketed with green grass and pockets of yellow daisies. You can feel the soft warm breeze brush against your skin and smell the sweet scent of pine.

➤ As you look up, you notice white, puffy clouds slowly drifting across a deep blue sky. Butterflies play tag against the faint sounds of birds twittering off in the distance. When you close your eyes, you feel yourself gently lifted onto one of the puffy clouds floating above the meadow. You're as light as a feather as you look below.

➤ Imagine yourself unloading all the stressors that you've been carrying around onto this cloud. Let go of any problems in your relationships, your latest work project, your biggest worry, problems you've been trying to solve. As you unload each burden one by one, feel yourself become lighter. Take all the time you need to unload.

➤ Then imagine as you leave the cloud that you're floating higher and lighter than before. Notice how it feels to be at peace without the things that distract you or bog you down. Savor that feeling. Continue floating with the clouds without your stress as long as you wish.

➤ When you're ready, imagine yourself being gently lowered back into the meadow beneath the shade tree. Notice how the grass feels against your skin. What sounds do you hear? What do you see and smell? You can continue resting here as long as you like.

➤ When you're ready, begin to bring your awareness back into the room. Notice that you are bringing with you a lighter feeling—a calmer heart and more relaxed body. Notice the seat beneath you and the sounds around you as your attention comes back into the room. Then open your eyes when you are ready.

Self-Created Visualizations

You can create your own safe harbor from stress by conjuring up feelings, thoughts, and body sensations that bring you calmness, peace and serenity. You can go to this inner refuge to become refreshed, relaxed, and recharged anywhere or anytime.

Bring up a positive memory or think of a person, pet, or spiritual guide that gives you comfort and joy. Or imagine your favorite place at the seashore or mountains. You could also create a place you've never been such as a secret garden or a place you've dreamed about. Here are a few other examples:

➤ A Caribbean island with waves lapping against your feet

➤ A Swiss Alps mountaintop with glistening snowflakes brushing your lips

➤ Swinging in a hammock in your own backyard with the smell of steaks on the grill

Focus on that image. See this place in detail in your mind's eye, creating item by item all the things around you that make this *your* personal haven. Notice what it's like to be in this place. Look around. What do you see? Listen. What do you hear? What do you smell? What do you feel? Name your positive emotions and body sensations as you hold in mind the image of this safe place.

Now, direct your attention to your internal sensory experience and notice what's happening inside. Note where in your body you feel the sensations that are pleasing to you. Notice the sensations in your breath, heart rate, and muscle tension. Bring your awareness to the changes and notice, for example, that your breathing might slow down or your muscles might loosen. Spend time underscoring whatever is the change. As you end, pay attention to your whole body and notice all the changes that have occurred since you focused on your refuge. Stay with that change for a few moments.

Recharging Your Batteries

You can write your own visualization, record it with soft music, and play it as often as you want. Or you can ask a friend to guide you through it. Appendix B shows you where you can purchase CDs of guided visualizations online. Or you can find them in most bookstores where music is sold.

After you have a clear vision of your refuge, savor your time there as long as you like. This is a place you can return to anytime you get stressed out. Before opening your eyes, make a mental note of it so that you can return as often and for as long as you like.

Meditation, Judgment, and Equanimity

Your judgment about a downturn in the economy, mounting bills, loss of a promotion, a faltering relationship, or fear of an upcoming job challenge creates more stress than the situations themselves. It causes you to suffer inside with worry, anxiety, or depression, magnifying the original situation.

Judgmental thoughts can easily overtake you no matter where you are—walking hand-in-hand at the seashore, playing catch with a child, or fishing with a friend. You don't realize when you're caught in a thought stream. Your family and friends and any kind of inner awareness become little more than vague, if pleasant, backdrops. In these instances, your mind uses you. When you practice meditation, you use your mind to navigate these types of stressful situations in a totally different way.

First and Second Zingers

Ever have an itch and the more you scratch it, the more it itches? Maybe you can't do anything about the itch, but you can do something about the scratch. Stress is a lot like that. When stress zings you, your reaction can add insult to injury, making you suffer worse. Your reactions to stress are second zingers—the ones you impale yourself with. The first zinger is unpleasant for sure, but sometimes the real distress comes from your second-zinger reaction instead of the stressful event. If you can avoid reacting when stress zings you, you can reduce your stress level.

Shock Absorber

When you fail at something, make a mistake, or have a setback, judging yourself creates a second layer of stress, making you more likely to give up. Facing an upsetting situation with impartiality reduces the intensity of your stress. Self-judgment throws you into a cycle of setbacks: "I ate a piece of carrot cake" spirals into, "I've already blown my diet now, so I might as well eat a second piece," which turns into, "I'm such a loser; I'll never get this weight off." It's not eating the cake that makes you feel bad; it's the second zinger (the stress you put yourself through) that makes you feel bad. The bad feelings throw you into a cycle of seeking comfort in the very behavior you're trying to conquer. When you remove the second layer of condemnation, you feel at ease to deal with the real stressor.

Suppose you hit your head on a kitchen cabinet. After the first zinger of pain, comes the second zinger of judgment: "Ouch! I'm such a klutz!" Sometimes second zingers trigger more second zingers through association. Maybe a friend is late for dinner (first zinger), and you feel your blood boil (second zinger). Your judgment of the situation brings up memories of abandonment as a child (another second zinger).

Sometimes you might have a second-zinger reaction when there's no first zinger to begin with. In these situations, your inner judgment creates stress by imagining there's a first zinger. Suppose you have a sinking feeling that an upcoming presentation to colleagues will go south before it even takes place. If you stop to think about it, the tension (second zinger) comes from an inner judgment (another second zinger) predicting you'll mess up. It's the self-judgment that distresses you; there is no first zinger.

Shock Absorber

This mindfulness exercise can help you stop second zingers in their tracks.:

Next time stress zings you, pay attention to your second zinger without judgment. A first zinger can be a stress-related body pain, an unsettling thought, or an upsetting situation. Note how many times you have a strong reaction such as lashing out, feeling bad inside, or both. If you are able to practice equanimity, note those times too. Then record your observations in your stress journal. See if you are able to observe yourself without judgment. If you discover that you *did* judge, see if you can refrain from judging yourself for judging.

Practicing Equanimity

When stress zings you, meditation helps you see the difference between the first and second zinger. As you develop the skill to see them as separate, you realize you don't have to react every time you get zinged. Known as equanimity, this distinction is good medicine for your stress level because it softens your reaction. In other words, you are able to be present with your mental reactions without reacting to them.

Stress Vocab

Equanimity is a meditation term that refers to the ability to stay calm amidst a distressful situation.

Attaining equanimity is not as easy as it sounds. Pulling it off is as difficult as resisting the urge to scratch an itch. And it takes practice. After practicing meditation for a while, equanimity can give you an inner feeling of separation from the urge to react. It lets you feel disappointment without suffering and frustration without acting out. It keeps you from adding more suffering on top of suffering.

How many times, for instance, have you been in the middle of an activity that required your full attention when someone interrupts you? Maybe you're irritated. The interruption is the first zinger and your irritation is the second zinger. Equanimity helps you recognize you're irritated but cushions you from the irritation so that you don't zing yourself again (in this case blow up).

Stressful first zingers can hijack your emotions and carry you away. But it's the second zingers that add another layer of distress. As you start to pay closer attention and bring self-compassion to your second zingers, you can greatly reduce your stress.

The Doctor Of Calm Is In

If you are distressed by an external thing, it is not this thing which disturbs you, but your own judgment about it.

—Marcus Aurelius

Meditation can help you recognize stressful states, transcend them, and still your mind. When you notice yourself in an unpleasant emotional state—such as worry, anger, frustration, or fear—focus on the feeling itself instead of pushing it away, ignoring it, or steamrolling over it. When you hold it at arm's length and observe it impartially as a separate part of you, you can prevent succumbing to it. Continue to welcome and observe the feeling nonjudgmentally with something like, "Hello frustration, I see you're active today." This simple acknowledgment and acceptance gets negative emotions to relax and calm down. My prescription: Welcome and observe stressful states of mind with curiosity instead of judgment as needed or until discomfort subsides. Here's to outsmarting your stress!

PART FOUR

Stress
and Your
Psychological
Health

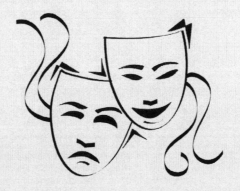

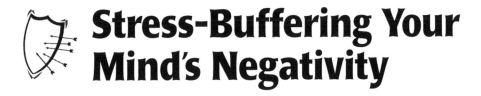 Stress-Buffering Your Mind's Negativity

In this chapter, you'll discover why your mind is wired with a negative slant that can stress you out. You'll get a better understanding of how easy it is to mistake imagined threats for real ones and how you can manage those situations. Plus, you'll learn how to prevent your negative expectations from contributing to stress and negative outcomes.

Why Your Mind Creates Stress

Let's start with why your mind creates stress and how that affects you. Then, we'll explore your part in managing these self-created stressors.

Your mind is designed to protect you at all costs. Mother Nature is more interested in marinating you in stress juices to keep you alive than in reducing your stress to make you happy. You have a built-in negativity bias that causes you to overestimate threats. You have an inner critic with beliefs and expectations that directs you in one stressful situation to the next. And as if that weren't enough, your mind filters the present through past experience so you won't make the same mistake twice (you'll only touch a hot stove once).

Truth Serum

Your mind creates stress even when none is present for one reason: survival. When a threat is perceived (real or imagined), you worry about it. Worry causes your body to respond as though the threat is real even when it isn't. And this activates your stress response. Much of the time you're stressed out more by imagined stress than real stress. That's because your mind is not willing to take the chance of missing a threat under do-or-die circumstances. It's thinking something like, "Make a mistake once, and I'm dead meat." So you're hardwired to err more on the side of safety than sorrow.

Tilt: Your Mind's Negativity Bias

Suppose your boss walks by your desk. You smile and nod. She looks straight at you, as if through steel, refusing to acknowledge your presence. You shrink inside, thinking you're in disfavor. Your heart races and you feel shaky. You worry about your job security. The next week the boss calls you into her office. Your stomach flip-flops. You tremble, but she smiles and gives you a glowing performance evaluation—confirmation that she doesn't hold you in disfavor but regards you as a highly valued team member.

Does this sound like you? Were you ever wigged out by an upcoming event and it turned out not to be a problem at all? If so, chances are your mind is trying to warn you with its negativity bias, which acts as an alarm system.

Stress Vocab

Negativity bias is the name scientists give your mind's built-in tendency to pay attention to and give more weight to negative versus positive experiences.

Mother Nature's Stress Proofing

The human mind is wired to routinely assess risks by making judgments about people and situations for protection. And negative experiences grab your mind's attention more than positive ones. If you're in a situation with a lot of information to pay attention to, you will immediately notice threats instead of opportunities. Forget the blooming azaleas along the roadside. If you don't see the car zooming at you at 90 miles an hour, you're roadkill.

Your mind constantly seeks pleasure and avoids pain. And it learns more quickly from pain than pleasure. You're more likely to store a negative memory after just one episode than a positive one. I'll bet you remember where you were and what you were doing on 9/11. But where were you the next week at the same time? You're more likely to remember the time you fell out of the tree and broke your arm than all those times you climbed the tree. Or that bad-tasting medicine your mom forced down you? You're more apt to remember that than her lemon meringue pie.

Do You Believe Everything You Think?

Because of the negativity bias, your negative thoughts are more automatic than positive ones. And you tend to believe them simply because you think them. "What about less stress and more happiness?" you ask. I imagine Mother Nature would respond with, "That's where your job comes in."

Fallout from your negativity tilt can take many forms, causing you to do one or more of the following:

➤ Accept negative comments and put-downs more easily and feel more comfortable with criticism than praise

➤ See the glass as half empty instead of half full

➤ Overestimate threats and underestimate possibilities

➤ Overlook the gains contained in your losses

➤ Allow one bad experience to rule your outlook in future situations

Although the negative tilt hardwires you for safety, it creates unnecessary stress, limits your possibilities, and keeps you from believing in yourself. To complete Mother Nature's work, your job is to go beyond survival thinking and avoid taking the bait every time a negative thought clobbers you.

Don't Bite the Hook

Imagine someone scolding you over your cell phone, and you hold it away from your ear. In the same way, you can hold a negative thought away from you and watch it from afar, without believing it or blending with it.

Think of a negative thought you've been carrying about another person, situation, or yourself. It could be something like, "I can't seem to do anything right lately" or "Going out with me is the last thing on her mind." Next, position yourself in a comfortable place, close your eyes, and watch the negative thought for a few minutes. Observe it as a part of you without judging it, just as you might notice a blemish on your hand. As you watch the thought, you realize it's not you and it's not necessarily true. You can observe your thoughts in this way without automatically believing them.

Recharging Your Batteries

Kayakers say the best way to escape when you're trapped in a hydraulic—a turbulent, funnel-shaped current—is to relax, and it will spit you out. But the natural tendency is to fight against the current. And that can keep you stuck, even drown you. Similarly, the way to get unstuck from a torrent of negative thoughts streaming through your mind is to welcome and watch them with curiosity. Let them come and go without personalizing them, resisting, or identifying with them. And eventually they float away.

Your Mind's Self-Talk

Have you ever had a sinking feeling before a presentation to colleagues or pitching an idea to management? If you stop to think about it, the feeling comes from an inner voice predicting you'll mess up or that your concept will not be received well.

Your Inner Drill Sergeant

You can't help forming judgments; that's how you make sense of the world around you. But as your mind overestimates threats, your self-criticism pumps up the volume, raising your stress level. Enter your inner critic—that kick-butt voice inside your head, telling you how worthless, selfish, dumb, or bad you are. Your inner critic is a part of your mind that constantly chatters away, expecting the impossible, never letting you rest. It uses negative self-talk, sounding like a drill sergeant who doesn't want you to get your head blown off in combat.

Stress Vocab

The inner critic is a critical part of your mind that points out your flaws and judges you harshly for your mistakes and failures, presumably to keep you on track.

Imagine you have your eye on a certain job for which you're qualified or that you're attracted to someone you'd like to ask out. But your fear blocks you from going after the job or the person. Your inner critic's judgments reverberate in your mind's echo chamber. You might be holding negative thoughts that you're unaware of such as you're unlikable, a failure, or not good enough.

When this happens, you're likely to think of the inner critic as you, to believe the imagined threat to be a real threat and avoid both scenarios to reduce your stress. There's no evidence for these beliefs. You haven't taken the first step to apply for the job or speak to the person you find attractive. But your inner critic warns you anyway so you don't get ridiculed or rejected.

Negative self-talk is self-defeating and stressful. When you fail at something or make a mistake, your disappointment is painful enough. But your inner critic adds insult to injury when it pipes up with thoughts of being a loser and amplifying your stress.

Your Inner Critic Isn't You

How many times have you felt torn about a decision? A part of you wants to go on a hike, but another part of you wants to be a couch potato. Just like a cake is a combination of ingredients—flour, milk, salt, sugar—you're a combination of sub-personalities, or parts. You can be forceful at times and yielding at others. Sometimes you're in the mood for a burger; other times you prefer a salad. The worry wart, perfectionist, and appeaser, discussed in Chapter 5, are examples of parts or sub-personalities.

Chances are your inner critic is one of your biggest sub-personalities. But it's not who you are, even though it sometimes feels like it. It's not present 24/7 and usually shows up when something big is happening in your life. When you're used to thinking of yourself in negative terms such as *lazy*, *rigid*, *unattractive*, *stupid*, *impatient*, *selfish*—the list is endless—it's the inner critic in you, not you.

Stress Vocab

A sub-personality is an aspect of your personality, or a part of you, that shows up on a temporary basis to help you cope in different situations.

Shock Absorber

When your inner critic overshadows you, remember: It is a stockholder, but you're the CEO. Your wrist is not you, your ribcage is not you—they are parts of you. There's more to you apart from your worry, apart from your perfection, apart from your doubt, apart from your judgment. Think of your inner critic as a separate part of you. Bring in the rest of you (your kinder side) to see the complete picture of who you are. And then let your self-compassion run the show, give you pep talks, and focus on the upside of situations.

Calling a Truce with Your Inner Critic

The Buddhist monk Thich Nhất Hanh told this story:

"Recently, one friend asked me, 'How can I force myself to smile when I am filled with sorrow? It isn't natural.' I told her to smile to her sorrow, because we are more than our sorrow."

Next time your inner critic pops up, try these tips:

➤ Realize your inner critic is speaking to you.

➤ Listen to your inner critic as a separate part of you, not all of you.

➤ Avoid arguing or trying to reason with your inner critic because it always has a comeback.

➤ Think of yourself as the CEO in charge of your mind's boardroom, and your inner critic as a stockholder. You can let it have an opinion without agreeing with everything it says.

➤ Use your kinder voice to run the boardroom and encourage and nurture yourself. Then, you're less likely to resort to self-sabotage.

Recharging Your Batteries

Do you reach for a quick fix to damp discomfort created by your mind's negativity? Do you procrastinate instead of address a problem, avoid unpleasant situations, or escape through addictions? If so, you'll notice that these self-defeating actions give you temporary relief in the heat of the moment. They feel like friendly solutions but are actually wolves in sheep's clothing that cause you more harm in the end.

If you're broke but want to go out on the town, stay home, have dinner, and watch a free TV movie. Then, you've reduced your debt. Spending money for a night out provides temporary pleasure but doesn't resolve your debt problem; it worsens it, and stress returns with a vengeance. So pay attention to your inner reactions to your negativity bias. And when attempting to soothe yourself, watch for self-sabotage. Make sure your actions are not short-term gain and long-term pain, but that they help and support you over the long haul.

Your Mind's Stress Road Map

Most people are not aware of it, but below their conscious mind they have more thoughts coming and going than Grand Central Station has trains. It's impossible to focus on them all or see everything around you at once. Your conscious mind is like a road map, restricting incoming information and narrowing its scope. This helps you focus on one thing at a time so you can understand the world around you and use prior experience as a safety scanner.

Try this experiment:

Ask a friend to take one minute and look around your office or whatever room you're in at the time. Ask the friend to list mentally as many items as she can that are blue—perhaps the carpet, wallpaper, bindings on books, curtains, and sofa.

When the minute is up, ask her to close her eyes and name out loud all the items she can remember that are yellow. Her mind will probably go blank; she won't remember yellow items because she was focused on blue. And she might squint at you and wonder if you've been sniffing the furniture polish.

As you can see, prior experience guides you so new situations make sense and you know how to respond to them. Problem is, sometimes old road maps can take you down the wrong road. Let me explain.

Getting Off Course

After a three-week trip to Southeast Asia, I returned to work unaware of having a new mind-set. I walked into a coworker's office and noticed a book on her sofa, only half of which I could see. I thought the title of the book was *Tea Ching* and believed that she too had an avid interest in Asian culture. Upon closer examination of the cover, I chuckled at the actual title: *Teaching in the Elementary School.* My Asian frame of reference caused me to bring a whole set of assumptions about this woman and her interests that were really about my experiences, not hers. My skewed beliefs (old road map) framed the situation incorrectly.

This small incident shows how your mind-set, formed from previous experience, governs how you perceive and deal with stress. Your past stress road map filters each current situation to keep you safe. It reminds you to lock your doors at night, to drive safely on the highway, to make sure you know someone before tying the knot, and to read a contract thoroughly before signing it. And it can create stress even when no stressor is present.

Translated into everyday life, what you experience or what you're taught to believe about yourself early on rules when you're grown. And it can cause you to make errors in judgment. For example, when you were five, you were bitten by a dog. At the age of thirty, your heart jumps into your throat when you see a dog off its leash. In childhood, you felt like you never measured up, and you freak out before the bar exam. You've had two heartbreaking romances, and you find yourself backing off from intimate relationships.

Much of the time your mind's reaction in the present is driven by past events that are no longer deadly or unsafe. In other words, your mind and body overreact to small things that create unnecessary and unpleasant stress in the present.

Been There, Done That, Got the T-Shirt

My own experience is a good example of how my upbringing served as a stress road map when I was in college.

I grew up in a poor family. As a child, I was self-conscious that I didn't have a nice house and clothes like the other kids. Once in college, unbeknownst to me, that less-than feeling had been housed in my mind to guide my actions. I was invited to parties and welcomed at social events, but rarely went because I thought of myself as an outsider. When I'd push myself to go, I'd unknowingly behave in ways that fit with my unworthy feelings. I avoided conversations and eye contact and stood on the sidelines to become invisible. Looking back, I can honestly say that I was smart and good-looking. But unbeknownst to me, my road map was directing me to avoid threatening social situations.

Shock Absorber

Describe your stress road map—your long-held beliefs from past experience that govern how you perceive and cope with stress. Jot down your thoughts in your stress journal. Then, see if you can think of times when your stress road map took you off course—when you overreacted to an imagined stressor that was driven by a past experience. Write those reactions in your journal. What information does this exercise give you that can help you manage stress in your current life?

Connecting the Dots with Murphy's Law

The lightbulb burns out in the bathroom, bedroom, and kitchen—all at the same time. Your TV is on the blink. Little things can make your life feel like it's falling apart. "Murphy's Law!" you scream. You rant. You rave. "If something can go wrong in my life, it certainly will." But is it Murphy's Law or your mind personalizing everyday random events?

The Science Debunking Murphy's Law

Actually, there's a science to all of this. You drop a piece of buttered toast and it always falls butter side down. Just your bad luck, you say? Not according to scientists at Aston University in Birmingham, England. After putting this question to the test, they found that buttered toast will almost always fall butter side down because of the law of physics. The rate of spin of falling buttered toast is too slow to make a complete revolution and come face up before it hits the floor. Not Murphy's Law at all, scientists conclude.

What about when you choose the slowest moving line at the supermarket? Murphy's Law you contend? Not according to scientists. The truth is that all lines move more or less at the same speed. Each will have its own delays that occur randomly such as the cash register running out of cash register tape or a customer who forgets a grocery item. Suppose there are three lines and you pick one. According to the law of averages, two-thirds of the time either the line to your left or the one to your right will move faster than yours.

Does Stress Feel Like a Personal Vendetta?

Those lightbulbs that all burn out at once were most likely installed at the same time and have a similar life expectancy. Chances are that the situations you write off as negative things that always happen to you have a scientific basis and have nothing to do with bad luck. So when you catch yourself overreacting to things not going your way, ditch that saying "just my luck" and remind yourself that the universe isn't against you and you're not jinxed. You're simply experiencing life's random events.

Recharging Your Batteries

When things go wrong, try not to personalize and magnify them into a negative life pattern. Chalk them up to the fact that things won't go according to plan from time to time and remember that it's the nature of things to break down, erode, and burn out. Learn to accept these situations as life's roll of the dice, not as a personal vendetta against you. You'll be less stressed out over the small stuff and less likely to develop a lifelong negative pattern of defeat.

Stress Vocab

A self-fulfilling prophecy is a belief or expectation, correct or not, that influences your behavior, which in turn produces an outcome that fits with your original expectation.

Shock Absorber

You can create positive outcomes the same way you create negative ones—by having positive expectations and behaving in ways that make them come true. When you can stay open to new experiences without making up your mind in advance, it works in your favor.

When was the last time you stuck your neck out? Start by identifying a stressor that has crippled or prevented you from living fully. It can be as small as learning to swim or balancing your checkbook. It can be as risky as facing a difficult relationship, dealing with a job loss, or launching into a new business venture. Find just one place in your life where you can stick your neck out and move through it. You will develop greater confidence and be that much closer to a stress-resistant life.

Stress and Expectations

You, like almost everybody, probably have certain expectations of how potentially stressful situations will play out before they happen. Usually, when you expect a situation to be a certain way, that's the way it turns out because you think and behave in ways that make your thoughts come true. This is called the self-fulfilling prophecy.

The Self-Fulfilling Prophecy

When you carry expectations around and superimpose them on an experience, it prevents you from seeing it for what it is. Your negative expectations create a mind-set of how a situation will unfold and how people will behave ahead of time. And you might not realize it, but you enter those situations with your mind already made up. Often when you expect a bad situation, it turns out that way because you think and behave in ways to make it fit with what you expect.

Suppose you're going for a job interview and a friend tells you that the interviewer is friendly, kind, and easy to talk to. No doubt you would go into the interview with an ease and calm that would be picked up by the employer. Your demeanor would give him a positive impression of you. This feedback would cause you to continue to present yourself in a favorable light that would probably get you the job.

On the flip side, suppose your friend tells you that the same man is a perfectionist grouch. He is hard to please and you would never be able to do anything right in his eyes. You would probably enter the job interview with a higher level of apprehension. You might forget to smile or appear nervous. The employer might sense your discomfort and form a negative opinion of you as lacking confidence or unable to function under pressure, making it less likely that you land the job.

Positive Expectations and Stress

Negative expectations bring you exactly what you bargain for: problems, discontent, and stress. The key to stress reduction is shifting your attitude from assuming the worst to developing strategies that yield positive outcomes. Here are some tips on how you can make the self-fulfilling prophecy work for you in a positive way:

➤ Underscore your triumphs and affirm your positive capabilities on a regular basis.

➤ Look for the silver lining in the cloud.

➤ Estimate threats and opportunities in balanced ways that keep you safe *and* foster your personal growth.

➤ Look for the gains contained in your losses.

➤ Learn from past mistakes and setbacks and see them as stepping-stones instead of roadblocks in the future.

Looking Through Fresh Eyes

Here's a true story that shows you how you can become aware of your negative mind-set, flip it around in a positive direction, and make it work to your benefit:

When I first set foot in Venice, I was dazzled by the beauty and culture—the aroma and flavor of Italian food, the priceless antiquities, the slope and design of the ancient buildings, and the romantic gondolas floating in the canals to the sounds of music from another time.

On the second day, I started to notice cracks in the pavement and buildings and how hot and dusty it was. The next day I noticed garbage floating in the canals and graffiti marring the buildings that I'd passed many times but hadn't noticed before. After a few more days, I'd had my fill of Italian food, and the music had become old hat.

By the end of the week, Venice had soured, and I was ready to bail. Then I realized it was my negative outlook—not the city—that had changed. Venice was still the same romantic, beautiful place when I left that it had been when I arrived. Once I flipped my negative outlook back to the same fresh eyes I'd looked through to begin with, the positive aspects gave me a complete change of heart.

The Doctor Of Calm Is In

I have been through some terrible things in my life, some of which actually happened.

—Mark Twain

When negativity clouds your outlook and creates stress, there's a lot you can do. How many times have you started a new job, project, or relationship, excited about the possibilities? Then over time you lose enthusiasm and your stress level rises. Maybe the situation didn't change— maybe your negativity bias kicked in and clouded your outlook. My prescription: Shift your negative perspective of an incident twice daily or as often as needed until positive feelings increase and stress symptoms subside. Here's to outsmarting your stress!

CHAPTER 15

 # Outwitting Stress by Changing Your Thinking

In This Chapter

➤ How your beliefs create stress

➤ ABCs of stress management

➤ Becoming aware of your stress-producing thoughts

➤ Avoiding mind traps

In this chapter, you'll learn to recognize the thinking filters that trap you in stress. You'll discover how to outwit stress by changing the content of your thoughts, challenging their beliefs, and testing new possibilities. Plus, you'll come away more mindful of how to dodge stress traps and balance your perspective in the future.

Psst, Look in the Mirror for Your Stressors

In the last chapter you learned one of the cruel facts of life: for good reasons, negativity has a longer shelf life and a more sustaining impact on you than positivity. Mother Nature left you and me to deal with stress fallout from the negativity bias. It's as if she says, "Okay, I've done my part to stress proof you. If you want to be happy, the rest is up to you."

By now, it's probably clear that to a large degree your perception of the world holds the key to your stress needle, and you have more control over your stress than you think, simply by the perspective you take. Here, I'll show you how to outsmart stress by challenging and changing your thoughts.

In the heat of the moment, it's easy to forget that your take on a situation causes stress. It's natural to look through your eyes, unaware of your thinking filter, and react based on that filter. And you write it off to external events—things like bills piling up, conflict with a coworker, an annoying salesperson, or misplacing your cell phone. Truth be told, the real stressor is not hiding outside of you but is in your own thoughts.

Don't Let Irrational Thoughts Stunt Your Growth

Imagine two passengers on an airplane preparing for takeoff. Neither one has flown before. Ann is so excited she can hardly stand it. Molly feels trapped, worries that the plane might crash, and stresses to the max. Ann listens to her iPod and relaxes. Molly white-knuckles it and grips the armrest during takeoff. Both have the same external experience but a completely different internal experience. Ann thinks about the flight as an exciting adventure. Molly believes something bad is about to happen.

What you say to yourself about a situation creates your mood, feelings, and reactions. And changing your thoughts gives you the tactical muscle memory to buffer stress. Let's look more closely at irrational thoughts.

Outfox Your Irrational Thoughts

You'll become clever as a fox once you realize that your thoughts are the real stressors. When you tune into what you say to yourself, the exaggerations become obvious. The more you listen, the clearer you become on how to change your thoughts. The first step is to recognize the irrational beliefs creating your stress. The next step is realizing you have the power to dampen stress by thinking about your stressors in a different way.

Shock Absorber

Increasing your level of emotional acceptance about a situation can help you outfox stress. The ability to accept change reduces the impact of stress. For example, Norma and June lose their jobs. Norma believes no employer will hire her at her age. She becomes angry, cynical, and defeated. Her hopelessness blunts her motivation, and she halfheartedly conducts a job search.

June believes regardless of her age she has a lot to offer an employer who can benefit from her skills. She quickly accepts being unemployed, eagerly launches a job hunt, and hooks two interviews within a week. June didn't let stress get the upper hand; she outsmarted it with her beliefs. And June isn't alone. Duke University researchers report that people who adopt an optimistic outlook are more likely to be quickly hired (more on optimism in the next chapter).

The ABCs of Stress

The ABCs of stress can help you stay calm when you feel like pulling your hair out. Suppose you're stuck in traffic, late for an important business meeting. You bang the steering wheel and explode, "Damn traffic! Now, I'll probably get fired!" You've just bypassed your perspective and blamed the situation. Plus, you've added a catastrophe that you have no evidence for. Truth be told, heavy traffic is just heavy traffic. It didn't happen to make your life miserable. It's your thoughts about the traffic that's causing you distress, not the traffic.

Once you start paying attention to the way you're thinking about stressful situations, it's amazing how it can change your reaction and lower your stress needle.

A Secret Formula for Sidestepping Stress

Psychologist Albert Ellis developed the A, B, C cycle to help you get a handle on how your irrational mind creates stress when you don't even realize it. Let's use his formula to plot your traffic scenario so it becomes clearer:

A + B = C

> ➤ A stands for the activating event, the stress trigger

> ➤ B stands for your belief or perspective about the stressor

> ➤ C stands for the consequence—your feelings and emotional reactions to the stressor because of your beliefs

In the traffic example, you jump from A (traffic jam) to C (freaking out, banging the steering wheel, and blaming the traffic) and bypassed B. Now let's go back and consider B (your belief), which is what creates most of C. Everybody has different beliefs about the events that stress them out. The key is for you to pay attention to yours. I'll plug in what some people might think in this situation, just to give you an example:

> ➤ A = Stuck in a traffic jam

> ➤ B = "Great, I'll be here all day long."
> "My boss will think I'm a slacker if I'm late."
> "Now I'll miss the meeting and probably get fired."

> ➤ C = Stressed and worried about being fired; angry at the traffic jam; automatic negative thoughts about work and the outcome of being stuck in traffic.

Challenging Your Exaggerated Thoughts

In the above example, you added insult to injury, because now you're not just stressed about being stuck in traffic (A), you exaggerate the situation by telling yourself you'll be here all day long and that you'll get fired for getting caught in traffic (B).

Much of the time, your beliefs in stressful situations raise your stress level because you believe the thoughts, even when they're exaggerated. Once you pay attention to what you're thinking and see how irrational it is, you feel calmer.

Shock Absorber

Think about some of the curveballs life has thrown at you and how you handled them. You probably remember the stressful event (A) and how upset you were (C). But you might not have paid attention to what you were thinking about the stressor (B). Here's a chance for you to go back and think about negative beliefs that could've contributed to your stress. Then, write down some positive thoughts that can mitigate the stressful feelings. I'll give you one example to get you started:

➤ Activating stressor: My computer crashed.

➤ Negative belief: "I'll never get this project in on time." Stress goes through the roof.

➤ Positive belief: "Computers sometimes crash. I'll find another way to finish the project." Calm prevails.

Changing Your Exaggerated Thoughts

Let's look at what you can change here. You can't change A because you're already stuck in traffic. But you can change B and C.

In the heat of a stressful moment, try to pay attention to your perception of the event. Once you're aware of your irrational thoughts, the next step is to change the way you're looking at the stressor. Tell yourself traffic jams are part of life and getting upset won't make traffic move any faster. It's highly unlikely that you'll be stuck all day and even more unlikely that you'll be fired for something beyond your control, especially since you're a loyal and highly productive employee (I hope I'm not exaggerating).

You can change C by reminding yourself that you have a choice of acting instead of reacting in this situation. You can choose to stay calm, people watch, or listen to soft music on your MP3 player or car radio. You can even capitalize on this time to do a body scan and relax different body muscles.

Next time, you might be able to change A by leaving earlier before traffic gets too heavy, taking a different route, or finding a different mode of transportation.

Recognizing Mind Traps

You can see how easy it is, without realizing it, to get swept away by negative patterns of thinking that distort the actual stressors in your life. What you say to yourself under stress pops up like burnt toast with such lightning speed that you don't even notice. Then you conclude that the external event is what upset you. Your stress is kept alive by the conclusions you make, many of which are inaccurate. You continue to draw wrong conclusions about situations because you keep falling into mind traps.

What Are Mind Traps?

Mind traps are irrational thought patterns that blind you to the truth, causing you to make errors in judgment about people, situations, and even yourself. For example, you might blame your anxiety on the fast pace of your job when, in fact, you overlook how your procrastination contributes. And you conclude the job is making your life miserable.

Stress Vocab

Mind traps are habitual ways of exaggerated thinking that cause you to draw illogical conclusions and over-personalize life events.

Identifying Your Mind Traps

Usually you're not aware that you're stuck in a mind trap, making a stressful experience more stressful than it has to be. Once you identify the traps you routinely fall into, it helps you manage your stressors.

Truth Serum

The cells of your body act like Mrs. Kravitz (from the TV sitcom, "Bewitched"), constantly eavesdropping on your thoughts, waiting in the wings to respond to threats. Suppose you're the nosy neighbor asked to give a talk at a community meeting. The first thought that pops into your head is, "I'll never be able to pull that off." (Burnt toast anyone?) Hearing this, your body's alarm system dumps cortisol into your bloodstream to help you deal with the stress. In a matter of seconds, you tremble at the mere notion of giving the talk. Your mind takes you out of the present moment, and in your mind's eye, a bloodthirsty audience of hundreds is staring you down. All the while your body is bereft with anxiety as if you're actually standing on the stage.

This mind trap is called catastrophic forecasting. It's an example of how distorted automatic thoughts can stew you in a stress soup, leaving you to wonder how in the world you got here from there to begin with.

Drs. Aaron Beck and David Burns identified common mind traps that you can get stuck in from day to day. Recognizing these traps heightens your awareness so that when you're trapped, you have an easier time escaping. Put a check mark by the following mind traps that snare you in your daily life:

➤ All-or-none thinking: "I can be either a good mom or a good employee; I can't do it all." You categorize life into the extremes of black and white and blind yourself to the shades of gray, where the truth usually lies.

The takeaway: Listen for yourself using words like *always, all, everybody, either-or, nobody, never,* or *none.* Let that be a cue that the all-or-none thinking has trapped you .

➤ Mindreading: "She didn't call me back. Obviously, I made a bad impression." You convince yourself you know what others are thinking and feeling. You connect the dots about a situation based on your beliefs, not the facts. When you automatically accept your thoughts as truth, instead of questioning or checking them out, you've sold yourself a bill of goods.

The takeaway: When you jump to conclusions in uncertain situations, remind yourself that your assumptions are not the truth. You can check out the facts before making conclusions to save yourself a lot of unnecessary worry and stress.

➤ Catastrophic forecasting: "I'm gonna fall flat on my face." You forecast the worst possible outcome of a situation without evidence for it. Even when facts contradict your negative belief, you continue to predict things will turn out badly.

The takeaway: When you catch yourself worrying over something that hasn't happened, identify your negative prediction. Then ask yourself, "Where's the evidence for this conclusion?"

➤ "Should" thinking: "I should have gone to church on Sunday." Oppressive words like *should, ought, must,* and *have to* shape how you feel about yourself. They can cause you to feel that you are slave instead of master of your emotions, leading to guilt, shame, and hopelessness.

The takeaway: Ask yourself if your self-talk opposes you or supports you. Replacing negative words with empowering words can change your feelings of being at the mercy of a situation to being in charge of it. Notice the different tone due to the replacement of one word in the following statement: "I could have gone to church on Sunday."

➤ Overgeneralization: "I really screwed up on that sale. I'm such a loser." You make a sweeping conclusion about your capabilities or worth on the basis of one negative event. You believe that if something's true in one case, it's true in all the others.

The takeaway: When you catch yourself viewing a negative event as a never-ending pattern of defeat, look at the proof. You'll likely not find evidence for the exaggeration. Remind yourself of your past successes.

Recharging Your Batteries

Next time you're caught in a mind trap, act instead of react.

Reacting is an automatic, defensive stance you take when your emotions govern your thoughts, and it allows you to be controlled by other people and situations.

Acting is a proactive stance that puts you in the driver's seat. When you pay attention to what you're thinking and then act, you use reasoning to deal with charged situations. See how often you can stay calm in a crisis, polite when someone is rude, positive when someone is negative. In each case, your thoughtful actions empower you to outsmart your stressors and turn the tone of a stressful situation around.

➤ Filtering and discounting the positives: "I won top broker of the year, but that was a fluke." You downplay your accomplishments or positive qualities and dwell on the negatives. This mind trap can keep you stuck in depression and anxiety and create an outlook of hopelessness.

The takeaway: There's usually a *but* in this mind trap that can help you catch yourself when you insist that your positive aspects don't count. Pay attention when negatives outweigh the positives and give the positives equal weight.

➤ Magnification or minimization: "I have to get this job promotion or my career goes down the tubes." You blow the negative aspects of a stressful situation out of proportion while shrinking your ability to overcome it. Or, on the flip side, you downplay your ability to surmount a stressful situation, "Oh sure, I got the last promotion, but that was because the boss liked me. I don't know the new boss."

The takeaway: Try to be aware when your outlook about a stressful situation is at one extreme or the other. Take the point of view of an outside observer and put it in perspective.

➤ Blame: "It's my fault the car broke down; I didn't take it in for service." You're overly responsible and blame yourself for conditions beyond your control. Or, on the flip side, you blame others, overlooking your part in an outcome, "I took your advice, and she broke up with me; it's all your fault."

The takeaway: Ask yourself if you're blaming someone for your actions. Then think about how much of the situation you're truly responsible for. Be willing to take ownership for your part, but avoid becoming overly responsible for situations outside your control.

> ➤ Emotional reasoning: "I feel hopeless about my marriage, so it must be over." You make judgments about people and situations from how you feel. And how you feel about something makes it true in your head, even if there's proof to the contrary.

The takeaway: Acknowledge your feelings first. Then see if you can separate them from the facts to determine if your conclusion is indeed true, "Yes, I'm feeling hopeless about our marriage, but that doesn't mean it *is* hopeless. There are steps we can take to make it better."

> ➤ Labeling: "I blew it with her; I'm such a jerk!" Instead of telling yourself that you made a mistake, you tell yourself you are the mistake. You put a negative label on people and situations because of one incident instead of looking at the entire picture, "I didn't like that movie; that theater sucks; I won't go there again."

The takeaway: Look at the big picture, "That *was* a bad movie, but that theater shows good movies, too."

Recharging Your Batteries

Think about the things you say to yourself right before, during, or after a stressful event happens. Answer the following questions in your stress journal:

> ➤ Which of the mind traps do you fall into the most?

> ➤ How do you overestimate the threat and underestimate your ability to cope with the mind traps you get caught in?

> ➤ What conclusions do you draw about the incident and yourself?

> ➤ Are your conclusions accurate, compassionate, and helpful?

> ➤ If you were on the outside looking in, how would you evaluate the conclusions?

> ➤ What would you say to a loved one who thinks this way about a stressful situation?

Getting Unstuck

As you can see, each of these mind traps is an exaggeration of a threat combined with an underestimation of your ability to deal with the threat. You'll remember from previous chapters that this is the way Mother Nature hardwired you.

Mind traps limit your possibilities and undermine the resources you have. They prevent you from seeing the truth about yourself by blaming you and leading you to feel helpless to cope with stressful challenges. They trap you into uncertainty and bad decisions, hampering relationships, and undermining progress toward your personal goals. But when you can step back and question your thoughts and conclusions, you automatically arm yourself with the ability to change your perspective and kick your stress-producing habit.

The Great Escape

When you get stuck in a mind trap, take the following steps for an escape hatch:

➤ Briefly describe the stressful event in a sentence. It could be a stressor you've had recently or one you're having now. Example: "I left out an important step in a big project."

➤ Write down the thoughts you have about the stressful situation that make you upset. Example: "My boss will be furious. We'll probably lose the account, and I'll probably get fired."

➤ Take your stress temperature based on your thoughts about the stressful situation using the 0 to 10 rating scale from Chapter 1. Example: "My stress temperature is a 9."

➤ Go through the list of mind traps and identify the one(s) you've fallen into. Example: catastrophic forecasting, overgeneralization, magnification.

➤ Once you realize how the mind trap distorts and exaggerates a situation, step back in your mind and substitute a more factual statement. Example: "I have no way of knowing what will happen, but in the past when I've made a mistake (which is rare), I worried about it. But it usually turned out better than I thought it would."

➤ Now take your stress temperature on the stressful situation again, this time based on your new outlook. Did your stress temperature drop? I bet it did. Example: "My stress temperature dropped to a 5."

Reeling in the What If's

One of the most common ways of overestimating threats is worrying about the future: "What if I'm not chosen for the position?" "What if I catch the flu before my party?" "What if the argument leads to a break up?" "What if there's a terrorist attack?"

*What if*s are exaggerated thoughts streaming through your mind that you latch onto as fact. You imagine the worst case scenario and play it over in your mind. But the truth is that most things never happen the way you imagine. Worry is a form of stress that interrupts your enjoyment of the present moment, keeping you stuck in a gloomy future that hasn't even happened yet. Your mind magnifies concerns about a situation and you end up stressing over a magnification of the problem, not the real problem. When *what if*s take over, they eclipse the truth about your capabilities to overcome challenges. And they factor out other possibilities at play that you have no knowledge of.

Most of the things you worry about never happen. Sometimes you have to wait for an outcome to convince yourself of an exaggerated forecast. Other times you can get a reality check from friends or coworkers. But the best stress-reduction technique is to suspend your *what if*s until you have convincing evidence. Staying open to the future and letting things happen instead of thinking about how they might happen can alleviate your stress.

When you wait to connect the dots after instead of before the hard evidence is in, you'll discover that *what if*s are unreliable sources of information most of the time. Finding the hard evidence first before jumping to conclusions saves you a lot of self-loathing, unnecessary worry, relationship problems, and time.

So, why worry? Ditch any unfounded beliefs before entering an uncertain moment in your life. And give the new job or relationship a chance to speak for itself before writing it off to *what if*s.

Shock Absorber

Here's how to turn foresight into 20/20: The next time a *what if* clouds your mind before an uncertain situation, intercept it and notice your internal reaction to the stressor. Think of yourself as a private detective and ask, "Where's the evidence for this conclusion?" You won't find any because there is none. Your evidence lies in hindsight. Think back to a few weeks or a month ago. Track some of the negative predictions you made about future events that have since happened. Write down some of the worries you had about a rained-out ball game, missing your plane, failing a test, or someone not liking you. Beside each negative conclusion, circle the worries that turned out the way you thought they would. Star the ones that turned out the exact opposite of your prediction. You'll probably have more stars than circles. When all is said and done, you won't find evidence for your worries; you're more likely to find evidence that contradicts them.

Finding the Middle Way

The next time a stressful event slams you and you start underestimating yourself, remember the lyrics from an old Eagles' song, "Already Gone":

"So often times it happens that we live our lives in chains / and we never even know we have the key".

The key is to recognize that it's not the situation that traps you but the way you think about and treat yourself in the situation.

Still, it's easy to get trapped by your mind's extremes and not realize it. It can feel like life is treating you badly when errors in perspective throw you on opposite ends of a scale, blinding you to the in-between, where actual truths and possibilities lie. Stress resilience doesn't come gift wrapped in black and white, magnification, or over-generalization. It's wrapped in shades of gray—that dot somewhere in-between the extremes known as the middle way.

Wearing Your "Graydar" Detector

The next time your mind gets stuck in extremes, here's a tool that can balance your thoughts and reduce your stress. I call it putting on your "graydar" detector.

First, make sure your antenna is up so you realize when you're snared in an extreme thought. Then draw a horizontal line across a sheet of paper. Write down your two extreme thoughts on each end of the scale. Then focus on the middle of the scale and write down other possibilities that exist in the shades of gray.

Here are a few examples:

> ➤ "I have to do the job perfectly (all) or I won't do it at all." (none) becomes "I don't have to be perfect in everything. I can take risks and learn from my mistakes."

> ➤ "If my husband doesn't read the self-help book, he's obviously not interested in making our marriage work." becomes "He doesn't have to read the book to do his part. There are many ways he can show his interest in working on our marriage."

The Doctor Of Calm Is In

The real voyage of discovery consists not in seeking new landscapes but in having new eyes.

—Marcel Proust

The lens of your mind—not your life conditions—determines your stress level. Once you see a situation from more than one standpoint, clarity heightens, stress drops, and inner peace of mind trumps the situation.

My prescription: Wear your graydar detector for the next twenty-four hours so you can see the blind spots that mind traps eclipse, or until you have 20/20 vision and you can see how you overestimate stressful situations and underestimate your ability to manage them. Continue wearing the device as needed to keep a balanced perspective and move your life in a positive direction. Here's to outsmarting your stress!

CHAPTER 16

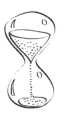

Stress Relief with Positivity, Optimism, and Self-Compassion

In This Chapter

➤ Building on positivity

➤ Broadening your outlook

➤ Recognizing your possibilities

➤ Cultivating optimism and self-compassion

In this chapter you'll discover how positivity offsets the negativity bias and acts as a stress buffer for mind traps. You'll find ways to broaden and build your positive outlook and develop optimistic strategies that make you more stress resistant. And you'll gain tools on how to use self-compassion to cushion stress and weather hard times.

Don't Worry, Be Happy

So far, I've discussed psychological stress health in terms of shifting your negativity bias and challenging and changing your thoughts. Here, I'll show you how positivity, optimism, and self-compassion relieve stress.

When negative emotions such as anger, anxiety, worry, fear, and hopelessness overtake you, they skew your understanding of the world. To say you're not going to worry—that you're just going to be happy—doesn't do justice to the scientific underpinnings of positivity's depth and power as a stress antidote.

As you'll see in this chapter, positivity, optimism, and self-compassion are powerful stress buffers. Let's start with negativity's counterpart, positivity. I'll show you ways to build on positive thoughts, emotions, and experiences. Then we'll move into optimism and self-compassion as stress antidotes.

The Downlow on Positivity as a Stress Buffer

One of the best-known positivity scientists Dr. Barbara Fredrickson at the University of North Carolina found that stretching your mind open to take in as much as you can creates positive outcomes. She and her colleagues assigned 104 people to one of three groups: group 1 experienced positive feelings (amusement or serenity), group 2 experienced negative feelings (anger or fear), and group 3 experienced no special feelings (neutrality). She then posed the question, "Given the feeling, make a list of what you want to do right now." The positive group had the longest list.

Truth Serum

Believe it or not, some scientists spend their entire careers studying the topic of positivity in the laboratory. Their research shows that positivity acts as a stress buffer because during stress it broadens the mind and range of vision. When you're threatened with a stressor, your mind is designed to constrict and target the negative threat. If you're searching for a solution to a crisis, your negative emotions keep you focused on the problem. Without knowing it, you focus on the stressful event and block out the big picture. But positive feelings like lightheartedness, joy, curiosity, gratitude, love, and hope expand your range of vision.

Positivity Showcases Possibilities

As you can see, a positive outlook leads you toward more possibilities than negativity or neutrality. When you're dealing with a stressful situation, positivity unlocks the range of possibilities. It helps you focus on a positive outcome that negativity hides from view. Simply put, negativity keeps you focused on the stress problem, and positivity helps you find solutions to problems you face in everyday life.

Stress Scope Quiz

Is your stress scope narrow or broad? The wider it is, the more stress resistant you are. To find out, answer how strongly you agree or disagree with the following statements. Then write in the number that fits: 1 = strongly disagree, 2 = disagree, 3 = agree, 4 = strongly agree.

____1. Life is full of problems.

____2. I usually assume people will take advantage of me.

____3. Things never turn out the way I want.

____4. Nothing I do is good enough.

____5. Whatever can go wrong will go wrong.

____6. I'm a born loser.

____7. Trouble follows me wherever I go.

____8. I'm not a worthy person.

____9. I can't change the way things are.

__10. I don't have what it takes to meet most challenges.

_____Total Score

Scoring: Add up the numbers and put your total score in the blank at the bottom. The lower your score, the stronger your stress scope is. Here's the breakdown:

10–20: You have a wide stress scope that makes you stress resistant.

21–29: You have a medium-width stress scope that you can build on.

30–40: You have a narrow stress scope that needs broadening in order for you to become more stress resistant.

Broadening Your Mind-Scape

As a result of many experiments, scientists say when you intentionally broaden your scope, your stress automatically lifts. A positive scope widens your attention, changes your outlook on life, expands your world view, and allows you to take more in and see many ways to buffer stress. The more you take in, the more ideas and actions you add to your toolbox.

There's a lot of wisdom behind the old adage, "Look on the bright side." Think about it this way: when a stressor hangs over your head like a cloud, you can't see through it, but creating positive feelings will help you part the cloudy thinking and the sun can shine through. As your scope widens, you see the big picture of possible solutions instead of being mired in the stressful event.

Harness Your Personal Resources

Do you blush when someone praises you? Do you feel like you pulled one over on someone who applauds your kind deed? Do you feel discomfort when someone compliments you on how you look?

There's a reason that *tallcomings* is not listed in wikipedia and *shortcomings* is. There's no such word as *tallcomings* because we ignore the positives and clobber ourselves with negatives. What about you? In a pinch, it's difficult to access your own positivity if you can't acknowledge the truth about yourself. Remember your job to complete Mother Nature's work is to broaden your perspective by finding your possibilities and personal resources. When you affirm these qualities on a regular basis, you have them at your disposal to overcome challenges in the future.

Recharging Your Batteries

It's important to recognize your limitations and failures. But don't drop your head in your hands. It's not as hopeless as you think. For an honest picture of who you are, it's also important to high-five your "tallcomings."

I bet you bend over backwards to build up the ones you love. But do you give yourself equal treatment, or do you go out of your way to bludgeon yourself with faultfinding? Naming the good things about yourself helps you see more of who you are. You can overcome a lot of stress by affirming both your strong points and areas for improvement by affirming your attributes and ability to overcome obstacles, and by treating yourself with the same kindness and consideration you give to others.

Throw modesty out the window and list all your tallcomings in your stress journal. Start each tallcoming with "I am.": *I'm smart, I'm strong, I'm resourceful.* Make your list as comprehensive as you can. Chances are your negative self-talk will object and try to block you. But be fair and honest. Think of your own positivity as a way to build your resources to face everyday challenges.

Broadening Your Positivity

Look over the list of negative statements in the Stress Scope Quiz. As you read down the list, notice the constrictive tone of the statements and how they cloud out possibilities. Notice how you feel as you complete the list. Not so hot, huh?

Now go back and broaden each statement to include possible solutions. For example, you might reword the first statement, "Life is full of problems," as "Life does contain problems and there are also solutions to problems; I can focus on the possibilities." After you've broadened the statements, notice the difference in tone. Do you notice a difference in how you feel? I bet you feel more uplifted.

Now it's your turn. Make a list of three or four negative thoughts you've had about yourself recently. Write them in your stress journal exactly as you hear them in your mind's echo chamber. Then go back and broaden the negativity by adding possibilities. Try to rewrite the statements genuinely in ways that are truthful for you. Pay attention to how you feel as you infuse more positivity.

Stacking Your Positivity Deck

It's simple science: when you feel positive emotions on a regular basis, they have cumulative benefits that trump your negative emotions. Scientists call this strategy the broaden-and-build effect. Here are some broaden-and-build strategies you can use to stack your positivity deck, blunt stress, and help you weather hard times:

> ➤ Step back from stressful events and brainstorm a wide range of possible solutions.

> ➤ Tell yourself stress is not a personal failure and that nothing is permanent. Every event has a beginning and an ending.

> ➤ Broaden your scope beyond the stressful event and think of the full range of things in your life that make you happy.

> ➤ Practice positive self-talk instead of making negative self-judgments.

> ➤ Dwell on positive subjects and focus on positive aspects of your life where you can make a difference. Avoid high-stress media reports, violent movies, or squabbles in the office.

> ➤ Hang out with positive people. Like negativity, positivity is contagious. When you surround yourself with positive people, positivity rubs off on you.

> ➤ Give yourself a fist pump when you reach a milestone or important accomplishment. Tell yourself how awesome you are: "I knew I could do it!"

➤ Focus on the solution, not the problem. Set realistic goals that help you cope with the stressor. For example, if you're dealing with trimming your budget, look for free fun activities, search for bargains and coupons, and find ways to earn extra money such as having a garage sale.

➤ Reframe gloomy prospects in a positive way. Few situations are 100 percent bad. If the weather forecast is 50 percent chance of rain, remind yourself there's a 50 percent chance it won't rain.

Recharging Your Batteries

If you're like many people, you automatically highlight the aspects of your life that make you hot under the collar: you have the same lousy job, the usual inconsiderate coworkers, or the party was nothing to write home about. You build up your negativity deck without knowing it, and that becomes the lens you look through.

You can trump your negative lens by learning to see and underscore the upside. Don't let pleasantness slip by without highlighting it. Start taking the pleasant aspects of the world into your mind: you love the way the breeze feels on your skin, you like how this tastes, or the smell of those flowers is wonderful. When you take the time to appreciate the smallest things around you, it cheers you up, grows positive feelings, and creates pleasing sensations inside you(such as slowed heart rate and softening of muscles) that offset stressful moments.

The Undo Effect of Positivity

Studies show that a positive outlook can undo the damage that stress and negativity do to your mind and body, making you more stress resilient. Positive events in your life help repair cardiovascular wear and tear caused by the stress response to negative events. Positive emotions send your body a different message than negative emotions, putting the brakes on the stress juices, activating your parasympathetic nervous system, and creating a calming effect.

Positive feelings contain the active ingredients that enable you to get away from debilitating stress and grow stronger. Positive thinkers are able to cope better with adversity because they can see solutions to stressful problems. Positivity helps you think *we* instead of *me*, to look past threats from people of different races, genders, or ages. Plus, it gives you an appreciation for the common ground you share with others. This broadening automatically draws you closer to friends and family. And you're more likely to feel at one with strangers, and people of different lifestyles, ethnic groups, and cultures around the world.

Shock Absorber

The gratitude exercise helps you see the flip side of things that stress you out. When you count your blessings, you broaden your outlook and lower your stress.

Write down in your stress journal as many things you can think of that you're grateful for, that make your life worth living. Then make a list of all the people, places, and things that bring you comfort and joy. Your list can include material items, such as cars, electronic devices, clothes, jewelry, houses, trips, and so on. It can include loving relationships, children, pets, and coworkers. And it can include your health and the health of your loved ones.

After you've made your list, reflect on your appreciation for each item. Practice this exercise regularly until you begin to see positive aspects of your life more often. You'll become more aware of how full life is instead of how much is lacking.

Optimism as a Stress Reliever

Tom was upset that he had to pay $500 thousand in taxes; he had lost count of the fact that he'd earned $5 million that same year. He was so caught up in his loss that it eclipsed his gain. Tom was a rich man living an impoverished life, all because of his negative attitude. Tom's attitude reminds me of something Benjamin Franklin once said: "While we may not be able to control all that happens to us, we can control what happens inside us."

Look for the Diamond in the Rough

Scientists say that when there is a flaw in a diamond, the diamond seems to lose its shine. Similarly, any hiccup in success makes some people feel like they're a failure. In graduate school, Lyn got upset when she made a course grade of A- and asked to take the final exam over in hopes of making an A+. To Olympians, gold is great but silver and bronze can be a disappointment.

Pessimism can be a knee-jerk reaction that you might not be aware of. A friend of mine loved the warm, long days of summer. One day in June on the longest day of the year, I said to her, "You must be on cloud nine." She replied, "No, I'm sad because tomorrow the days start getting shorter again." When I pointed out how she was shrinking her joy, she was unaware and surprised that her negativity had hijacked her. She was able to broaden her outlook, remembering how she'd looked forward to this time of year, and savor the warm weather instead of focusing on the cold days to come.

Trending Now from the Smart Files

Here are some ways that optimism can pay off:

> ➤ New sales personnel with an optimistic outlook sell 37 percent more life insurance in their first two years than pessimists.

> ➤ Students do better on standardized tests when they produce positive feelings during test taking. And children have higher gains in school achievement when teachers have positive expectations of them.

> ➤ Optimists scoot up the career success ladder faster and farther than pessimists.

Optimism Expands Your Contentment

Evan considered other people's accomplishments as his own personal failures because he hadn't reached the same pinnacle. When you use someone else's life as a yardstick to evaluate your own, you judge yourself unfairly and come out on the short end of the stick. This caused Evan to overlook his own triumphs that those he envied hadn't achieved.

Are you living the life of an underdog, or are you living at the top of your game? What you think about and focus on expands in scope. Lack creates more lack. You might feel as if your life sucks, despite the fact that others think you have a charmed life.

On the flip side, wanting what you have instead of having what you want creates more self-acceptance, life satisfaction, and stress-free living. Scientists say that optimism literally expands your peripheral vision and lets you see more than you usually do. It shows you who you truthfully are, the personal resources you have, and the opportunities embedded in stressful conditions.

No wonder studies show that optimists have lower stress levels and more stable cardiovascular systems. You can also see why blood samples reveal that optimists have stronger immune systems and fewer stress hormones than pessimists. Optimists know and believe in their capabilities and adopt healthier habits, too. Statistics show that optimists have fewer health complaints, healthier relationships, and live longer than pessimists.

Truth Serum

Statistics show that on average optimists live seven and a half years longer than pessimists. One research study of 2,800 heart patients reported that those optimistic about their heart disease were more likely to live fifteen years longer than those with a pessimistic outlook. Heart patients pessimistic about their condition were 30 percent more likely to die during the study period. And Dutch scientists report that the death rate of optimistic men is 63 percent lower than their bellyaching peers; for women, optimism reduced the death rate by 35 percent. Long live the optimists!

Turn Your Life Around with Optimism

Optimists don't possess some magical joy juice. They're not smiley-face romantics looking through rose-colored glasses. They are realists who take positive steps to cope with stress rather than succumb to it. It might be difficult at first for you to find the diamond in the rough. But you can gain a lot by cultivating an optimistic outlook. And it gets easier with practice.

Think about it. Being able to see the positive side of a negative situation can arm you with the hope of overcoming obstacles you face. So practice looking for the silver lining in situations you perceive as negative. Even if your life is stressful, find one or two positive things that you enjoy and look forward to. Surround yourself with optimists instead of pessimists who pull you down. Pay attention to the attitude you bring to work or home and try to keep it in check.

In a pinch, your mind-set tends to fall on the negative side. But you can ask, "Is the glass half empty or half full?" See the gains in your losses, the beginnings contained in your endings. When you hit forty, you can think of it as half a life left or half a life lost. When you enter a rose garden, you can savor the beauty and fragrance of the flowers or feel repelled by the thorns. You can usually find a granule of good in the bad when you look for it.

Peek at Stress Through Your Wide-Angle Lens

Like the zoom lens of a camera, the mind zeros in on stressful situations, magnifying problems and hardships and eclipsing the big picture. Once you understand that positivity is always present even when you're under stress, you can start to focus your mind more on the upside and build on it. Try using these steps to shine a different light on stressful conditions:

> ➤ Pinpoint the challenge or opportunity contained in each negative experience.

> ➤ Empower yourself. Remember the personal resources you have at your disposal to overcome the event and how the stressor provides an opportunity for you to learn more about yourself.

> ➤ Take the viewpoint that mistakes and stressful situations are lessons for you to learn (open-ended curiosity), not failures for you to endure (close-ended judgment). Ask yourself what you can learn from the stressful event so that you'll be more resilient next time.

> ➤ Turn the stressor around by focusing on the opportunity it contains. Ask yourself: "How can I make this situation work to my advantage?" or "Can I find something positive in this negative situation?" or "What can I manage or overcome in this instance?"

See if you can make it a goal to use each experience—no matter how stressful—as an opportunity to get to know your inner strengths and become more stress resilient.

Shock Absorber

Do you look at life through a zoom lens or is yours a wide-angle lens? One way to find out is to identify a complaint you have about something. Perhaps your mutual fund isn't worth as much or you worry that you have to pull several all-nighters to get caught up at work. Once you recognize a complaint, put on your wide-angle lens by pulling up the big picture, seeing the complaint in the scheme of your whole life. As you broaden your outlook, how important is the judgment you've made against your life or yourself? If you're like most people, the complaint loses its sting when you put it in a wider context.

Look for the Gift in a Cosmic Slap

Actor/comedian Richard Belzer once said, "Cancer is a cosmic slap in the face. You either get discouraged or ennobled by it." In a Barbara Walters interview, actress Elizabeth Taylor said she laughed when doctors told her she had a brain tumor. Walters gasped. But Taylor wisely replied, "What else are you going to do?" Actually Taylor's and Belzer's attitudes prove you can do a lot when adversity strikes.

If you're not a natural-born optimist, no worries. You can learn coping skills to face the seismic events in your life. The main skill is to discover the gift in adversity. Then focus on how that gift changes your life for the better. In referring to the motorcycle accident that paralyzed him, Sean said, "It was probably the greatest thing that ever happened to me." The accident changed Sean in ways that otherwise would not have been possible. Recovering alcoholics often say hitting bottom is their greatest blessing because it wakes them up to a brand-new way of living. After grieving the heartache of a broken relationship, many people say they find healthier, more meaningful relationships.

The meaning in your cosmic slaps can enrich your life if you're willing to look at it that way. Studies of trauma survivors show that adversity can have the following benefits:

➤ Help you see you're stronger than you thought

➤ Bring new meaning to your life

➤ Take you deeper into your spirituality

➤ Deepen the closeness you feel to yourself and others

An amputee from the Iraq War counsels other disabled soldiers. A person with HIV volunteers time to help raise money for AIDS research. Adversity's biggest gift is helping you see your inner fortitude and ability to find richer meaning, which you might not have otherwise known was there.

Self-Compassion: A Powerful Stress Antidote

If you're like many people who kick themselves around for their shortcomings, you probably have a deep belief that this treatment can help you do better. Or you might worry that giving yourself too much leeway might turn you into a total slacker. Truth be told, negative self-judgments actually increase your stress, whereas compassion is a more powerful stress-resilient tool. Studies show that when you substitute self-compassion for self-criticism, you foster positive change in just about anything you do.

Stress Vocab

Self-compassion is the kind, supportive treatment you give yourself each step of the way during personal shortcomings, challenges, and setbacks.

Hard Evidence for Self-Compassion

Scientists say self-compassion stops worry, fear, and other negative feelings in their tracks. When you're self-compassionate, you don't deny the hardships you're going through. You admit the pain, suffering, fear, or whatever you're feeling. Then, you emotionally support yourself through the struggle instead of turning on yourself or putting yourself down in the middle of it.

Put Down Your Gavel

You, too, can cultivate more self-compassion and stop stress cold in its tracks. After you have a setback, self-condemnation often barges in. But the real stressor is self-judgment, not the setback.

Truth Serum

Dr. Kristin Neff at the University of Texas examined self-compassion in the laboratory. She found that when you're hard on yourself, it's more difficult to bounce back after a setback, and you're more prone to anxiety and depression. But when you replace negative judgments with self-compassion, you recover more quickly. And if you don't have self-compassion, no worries; you can develop it. After an eight-week program of mindfulness-based stress reduction (composed of yoga, meditation, and relaxation exercises), 90 percent of Dr. Neff's participants increased their level of self-compassion.

You'll remember from Chapter 13 that when you remove the second layer of judgment (the second zinger) and substitute compassion, you can see the stressor (the first zinger) more clearly and feel more at ease dealing with it. That's why it's important to be gentle and supportive with yourself when you're under the gun. So start wanting only the best for yourself in everything you do. Above all, be willing to catch yourself when you fall just like you would for a best friend.

Use Comforting Self-Talk

You wouldn't dream of treating a loved one the way you treat yourself: calling yourself names, pelting yourself for the smallest human mistakes, disbelieving in yourself enough to give up on your goals. When you're feeling sad, in pain, or grieving, harsh words such as, "Stop feeling sorry for yourself," or "There are people worse off than you," or "Get a grip!" can actually worsen your stress. But a compassionate voice with a calming, comforting tone helps you cope as if you're applying salve to a wound.

Self-soothing is especially beneficial in the aftermath of such stressors as separation, divorce, job loss, natural disaster, diagnosis of a serious illness, or death of a loved one. Pep talks and supportive words are especially beneficial in the middle of high-pressured situations such as life-and-death emergencies, job interviews, performing in front of your peers, competing in a sports event, testifying in a court case, and so on. So whether you're dealing with a big crisis or small hassles, a kind, nurturing voice spares you a lot of stress, calms you down, and carries you through to its end.

Talk Yourself Off the Ledge

Under duress, it helps to imagine you're embracing a distressful emotion with soothing words. Here's an example of how you could tenderly whisper to your emotion just as you would to a child or loved one:

Dear One,

Things are tough right now. That sucks and it brings up a lot of unpleasant feelings. If I could take the hurt away, I would in a heartbeat. But I want you to know you're not alone. I care about you and am here with you. I'll stay close to you every step of the way. No matter what happens, I'm right here with you, and we'll get through this together.

During emergencies or high-stress situations, you might use a firmer, peppier tone to convey a more reassuring message to your distressful feelings. For example, I got caught in a harrowing blizzard in a remote area of the mountains without snow tires or four-wheel drive. I couldn't stop or pull off the road, and my car was skidding on the ice. Clutching the steering wheel, I had to drive another 30 miles to civilization. So I took a deep breath and cheered myself on with something like this:

Okay, easy does it. You're doing great. You've got this in your pocket. Geez, you've handled a lot more challenging situations than this. And you've come out on top. You're going to be just fine. That's it, no rush. Just breathe and take your time. That's right, just keep it on the road. Awesome job!

Although the situation was stressful, nurturing myself through the frightening experience boosted positive feelings within me. The care and comfort I felt alongside the fear softened my stress level and helped me believe in myself. It reminded me that I'm resourceful, kept me calm, and helped me cope. Needless to say, I made it through without a scratch. But what if I'd spoken harshly to myself during the crisis? If I'd said something like: "You dumb ass! Why didn't you check the weather forecast before you left?" I'm not sure I'd still be here to write this book.

Recharging Your Batteries

Dr. Neff's research explains why self-compassion soothes your stress: not because you replace negative feelings with positive affirmations but because as you embrace your negative feelings, new positive emotions rise up within you. So find ways to embrace instead of replace your negativity. Taking your own side and talking to yourself in kind, supportive ways calms you down when you're upset and helps you get through stress. So next time stress hits home, talk to yourself in endearing terms that help you cope instead of in harsh words that make you feel worse and undermine your coping ability.

Be Kinder to Yourself

The main takeaway here is to separate yourself from your shortcomings and see them for what they are: habits, old behavior patterns, or just plain mistakes that all of us make. If you're kinder with yourself and accept your limitations with compassion, you cut your stress in half. Then you're dealing only with the stressful experience, not the added negative feelings from self-judgment.

Start to watch how often you put yourself down, call yourself names, or shame yourself with words like *should*, *ought*, or *must*. In your stress journal, make a list of the times you berate yourself. Then start to stand up to the impossible standards and harsh judgments instead of attacking yourself. Your nurturing voice can use objective information such as compliments, affirmations, and positive feedback from friends, coworkers, and loved ones. As you self-soothe, throw flattery out the window and be fair and factual.

If you'd like to know how kind you are to yourself (as if you didn't already know), you can go to Dr. Neff's official website, www.self-compassion.org/test-your-self-compassion-level.html and take her Self-Compassion Scale. After taking the test, a program will calculate your score.

The Doctor Of Calm Is In

We free ourselves from the prison of trance (unworthiness) as we stop the war against ourselves and, instead, relate to our lives with a wise and compassionate heart.

—Tara Brach

Studies show that when you're self-compassionate, you free yourself from negativity. You have more positive emotions such as enthusiasm, interest, inspiration, and excitement than self-critical people have. And you're more stress resilient and confident about meeting daily pressures. Winston Churchill said, "A pessimist sees the difficulty in every opportunity; an optimist sees the opportunity in every difficulty." My prescription: Each time you're under stress, put on your wide-angle lens and look for possibilities and opportunities. When you find opportunity by underscoring the upside in difficult situations, you'll feel better in twenty-four hours. Smiley face not required. Here's to outsmarting your stress!

PART FIVE

Managing Stressful Conditions in Your Life

CHAPTER 17

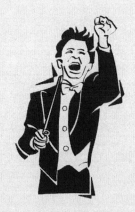

De-Stressing Your Personal Surroundings

In this chapter you'll learn field-tested ways to eliminate environmental stressors, get organized, de-clutter your surroundings, and establish a stress-free atmosphere. Plus, you'll discover simple and inexpensive ways to transform your personal areas into a soothing escape from the pressures of the day.

Environmental Stressors

It's hard to believe, but your everyday surroundings can keep you in a state of low-grade stress. And chances are you've become so used to clutter, noise, harsh lights, and other environmental stressors that you don't even notice they're making you feel stressed.

Studies show that under environmental pressure, your stress hormone levels can escalate even when you're not aware it. But over time, these hormone levels take a toll on your mental and physical health. This section describes some environmental stressors to be on the lookout for and how, where possible, to take steps to alleviate them.

Noise Pollution

TV or radio blaring reports of war, murder, robbery, and other tragedies, and commercials for headaches and acid relief are constant reminders of stressors you're probably trying to escape from. But are these intrusive broadcasts blaring in the background of your personal space? Plus, lawn mowers, car engines, and loud music increase stress levels and interfere with your serenity. Do outside noise polluters jar your peace of mind? Scientists say that steady exposure to loud noises such as traffic, aircraft, and railway engines raise stress levels that can lead to high blood pressure and fatal heart attacks.

If you're surrounded by noise pollution, consider muting jarring news events. Soundproof outside racket as much as possible with insulation, window treatments, pleasant background music, nature sound machines, headphones, or earplugs.

Air Pollutants

Cigarette smoke, chemical smells, mildew, toxic odors, and air quality—all can raise your stress level and lead to illness.

To help counteract air pollution, maintain a well-ventilated space with as much fresh air as possible. Use humidifiers in dry areas and dehumidifiers in humid places. Ban tobacco smoke from your personal space.

Trending Now from the Smart Files

Here are some stats on stressful environments:

➤ A 2011 National Sleep Foundation report said that one in five people say they are awakened at least a few nights a week by a cell phone call, text message, or e-mail.

➤ According to a *New York Times*/CBS News poll, 30 percent of those under age forty-five said the intrusiveness of electronic devices increases stress levels, making it harder to focus.

➤ Researchers at Minnesota State University found that people waiting in red-colored rooms had higher stress levels than those in green-painted rooms.

➤ Cornell University researchers found greater stress hormone levels (adrenaline) among people exposed to low-level noise compared to those exposed to quiet surroundings.

Light and Temperature

Artificial lighting is a subtle form of environmental stress, and limited sunlight can trigger depression and elevate stress, more for some people than for others. Rapid temperature changes also can trigger stress. And room temperature that is too hot or too cold can interfere with your concentration and escalate tension.

To enhance your environment, create a well-lit space while avoiding harsh lights. Use indirect lighting and as much natural sunlight as you can harness. Consider installing dimmers to control brightness and to create a soft, relaxing mood.

Mess that Leads to Stress

Disorganized and cluttered living spaces can make your life chaotic and stressful. Clutter becomes a roadblock to finding things you need, cutting into valuable time, and adding another level of frustration when you're in a hurry. As things pile up, your stress level can go sky-high. You might find your productivity wanes as you bounce from one task to another, paralyzed by where to begin.

After a long day when you're trying to relax, the last thing you want is stressful visual reminders of what needs doing staring you in the face. If you're like most people, you're looking for visual rest. De-clutter by deciding what you really need and what you don't. Then toss, donate, or recycle.

Shock Absorber

It pays to have a system and get in the habit of using it to eliminate unnecessary stress. An organized system for electronics, keys, mail, and other personal belongings eliminates the pressure of searching when you're already in a hurry. When your personal space is uncluttered, visually appealing, and functioning smoothly, your life is calmer.

There's something freeing and peaceful when things are in their place, the kitchen bar is free of junk mail, and dishes are off countertops and stacked in cabinets. Order conveys a feeling of calm and stability—a feeling that things are under control and all is right with the world.

Getting Organized

If you're like many people, when you get home, your mind is on powering down; it's not on where you placed your cell phone, keys, mail, and work tools. But when you can't find them, you spend precious time and needless frustration backtracking.

Wouldn't you much rather come home to a soothing refuge that helps you unwind—an orderly, well-organized space that evokes pleasant memories, feelings, sounds, and smells? A restful, stress-free atmosphere provides a stability and security that neutralizes the pressures of your day and gives you feelings of tranquility.

Take a Stress Inventory of Your Surroundings

Ask yourself if your personal surroundings are stressful or soothing. If they're stressful, there's a lot you can do to dig out from under the pile, get organized, and create a stress-free space.

For starters, take an inventory of your personal environment. Rate where the stress needle falls on a scale from 1 to 2: low stress, 3: medium stress, 4 to 5: high stress on the following conditions:

➤ Environmental stressors

➤ Organization

➤ Physical room arrangement

➤ Sensory comfort

➤ A touch of nature

➤ Lighting

Devising Your In-Home Stress-Reduction Plan

As you read on, devise a plan to lower your stress needle from a 4 or 5 on each condition to a 1 or 2. Let's say, for example, that you rate room arrangement a 4 because you have a sofa against a large window blocking a wooded view with a bird feeder. Part of your in-home stress-reduction plan could be to position the sofa so that the view brings more nature into your personal space. This action might lower your stress needle to a 2. Record your stress-reduction plan in your stress journal.

"Shovel Ready" to Dig Out from Clutter

When you're ready to de-clutter, you can start digging out with an inventory of personal belongings. Get rid of as many unusable items as you can. As you go along, organize them into four action categories:

➤ Keep: Whatever you keep make sure it has its place.

➤ Trash: Toss as many items as possible, especially those you haven't used in over a year that are not worth recycling or donating.

> ➤ Recycle: Keep a recycling bin close by.

> ➤ Donate: Have a special bin for donations for Goodwill, Salvation Army, or a yard sale.

These four categories give you set actions to help you make decisions and avoid getting bogged down by uncertainty.

Organize the Keepers

Use storage bins and organizers in your garage or attic to order the items you decide to keep. Install shelves and organizers in as many spaces in your closets and storage areas as you can to maximize the most of your space, keep things orderly, and eliminate frustrating searches.

Shock Absorber

Consider the rule that as you accumulate something new, you keep clutter down by getting rid of something old. This rule can keep you honest with yourself when it's hard to part with your "little darlings," the keepers you've held on to that you promised you'd use and haven't. Fess up about that ten-year-old toaster you've been keeping in case the new one fizzles out, the stack of magazines from the 1990s, the dinosaur computer that they don't make parts for anymore, or the melted candle you never relit and stored in the attic for the last two years. Need I go on? I'll bet your Keep category is shrinking by the second.

Create a Communication Hub

A central station in your kitchen or den can help you organize the avalanche of junk mail, important bills, fliers, doctor's appointments, prescriptions, coupons, kids' permission slips, catalogs, magazines, and newspapers.

Install separate plastic wall racks so that all household members have slots for their papers. Mount a bulletin board with announcements, brochures, and a large scheduling calendar that provides at-a-glance reminders of who needs to be where and when. You can use a different color pen for each family member so that a quick glance shows what pertains to whom.

Have a small desk with a computer, phone, and container for pens, pencils, paper, stapler, tape, and sticky notes for quick reminders. Beside the desk, place a small file cabinet for important papers and documents. Consider an attractive pottery bowl for business cards. The next time you need an electrician, plumber, or carpenter, their contact information is at your fingertips.

Sort incoming mail into separate inboxes for junk mail and important mail and a separate outbox for outgoing mail. Keep a recycling bin and trash can nearby your station so that junk mail, used envelopes, old catalogues, and outdated magazines or phone books don't pile up and clutter your space. Designate special hooks for keys and slots for coupons. Create compartments for cell phones, iPods and other devices so that your gadgets are easier to access and keep up with.

Follow the OHIO Rule

Clutter often exists because you can't decide what to do with things as they accumulate. So you do nothing. Items get shuffled around, time passes, and your piles, closets, shelves, and storage areas start bulging at the seams. The acronym OHIO (only handle it once) can be an efficient and time-saving tool to help you de-clutter your paper mail, e-mail, voice mail, and household storage areas.

The rule is either make an immediate decision about where something belongs or discard it. This rule prevents you from falling into the trap of moving junk mail or garage items from one pile to the next over and over again. You can also apply OHIO to deleting voice mail and spam e-mail right away instead of reacting to it and coming back to it later to refresh your memory. The result is a tidier inbox for your voice mail, e-mail, and paper mail, and added time to tackle more important tasks.

But OHIO might not always be practical or possible. All things don't lend themselves to snap decisions. You might be uncertain about some items and need more time to mull them over. But if you're in serious need of de-cluttering, OHIO can be an efficient rule to apply.

De-Clutter Your Paper Trail with Electronics

One way to de-clutter is to sign up for online billing. You can have paychecks automatically deposited, pay bills online, or have payments automatically deducted from your accounts. With electronic billing and payment, you eliminate excess mail and paper clutter. Plus, you save postage and the time it takes writing and mailing checks. You also eliminate your paper trail by electronically sending your grocery list to your smartphone. Plus, you can text or e-mail messages to other family members instead of writing them down.

Shock Absorber

Is all this talk about order and organization stressing you out? If so, take a breath and step back. Getting your personal space into stress-free shape can be overwhelming. If that's true for you, consider hiring out if you can afford it. The payoff of having a professional organizer, cleaning service, handyman, plumber, or gardener to get your home up to speed might be worth the expense in the long run.

Another option is to engage a friend or family member to assist you. An outside observer is less attached to your personal belongings and can give you objective tips on "when to hold 'em and when to fold 'em." There's usually one in every group dying to organize, arrange, and design someone else's stuff.

Take it One Step at a Time

If you have a lot of de-cluttering and organizing to do, make a list of the different spaces you want to focus on. Then take each area one at a time so you don't get overwhelmed.

At this writing, I have an upstairs kitchen closet in disarray and a downstairs junk closet and basement that need organizing. My plan is to focus on the kitchen closet first and keep everything else out of the picture. That plan keeps me from getting sidetracked by other places calling for my attention.

Before tackling the space, take a deep breath and give yourself plenty of time to finish. Once you get one area of your home tidy, you're more likely to pick up steam to start with the next one.

Stress-Free Room Arrangement

Everybody's personal space is different. When all is said and done, it's up to your creativity, imagination, taste, and unique schedule that determine how you de-stress, arrange, and decorate

Recharging Your Batteries

If you work at home, confine your work space to a specific area so that your projects don't intrude into the lives of other household members or constantly remind you of what you have to do. Refrain from spreading work out on the kitchen table or checking e-mails, voice mails, or texting while watching TV in your den.

Even if you live alone, after a reasonable day's work put away your electronic devices just as you would store carpentry tools after building shelves or baking ingredients after making a cake. Keeping work reminders out of sight keeps them out of mind and helps you relax and recharge your batteries.

your physical environment. In this section, I've hit some of the highlights that you might want to keep in mind as you go.

Recharging Your Batteries

Consider stress proofing your workstation by personalizing your office. During the pressures of the day, a pleasant work space can ease stress, help you stay calm, and improve work performance. Office photos of my dog and with friends on African safari warm my heart and lift my spirits at a glance. In addition to photos of pets and loved ones, bring in nature with plants and flowers. Block excess noise with earphones or soft music if allowed. Sounds of a small waterfall or the smell of a scented candle can aid relaxation. And, of course, keeping your work area as organized and tidy as possible also helps reduce stress.

Common Ground and Private Areas

Your best friend might think blasting Lady Gaga's latest CD is the coolest way in the world to unwind. But to you, it could be the most stressful activity on the planet. Personally, I adore Lady Gaga, but that's neither here nor there. The point is that what's environmentally stressful for one person might not be perceived as stressful for someone else. It's all in how you look at it.

So when planning stress-free zones, it's important to keep in mind that there's no one-size-fits-all solution. Some people tolerate more clutter and disorganization than others. You might prefer to have a little "comfort clutter" so that everything around you isn't so properly arranged that you feel like you're living in a museum. Or you might be a neat freak who is more at ease with surroundings that are pared down, tidy, orderly, and streamlined.

If you live with others, be considerate of the environmental stress thresholds of each household member. Agree to certain common areas that are maintained to suit everyone's needs. Separate personal areas such as bedrooms or office spaces can be individually maintained based on unique schedules and personalities. Whether you own or rent a house, condo, apartment, or cabin in the woods, planning for individual personalities can save a lot of animosity and promote emotional harmony among family members and housemates. So make it a win-win for everybody concerned.

Designate a Stress-Free Zone

No matter how frantic your schedule, you can always take time out to decompress. Having a special place to relax makes you more likely to hit your pause button.

Assign a getaway in your home, where you're not allowed to think about, feel, or deal with stressful issues. Make this stress-free zone a place of solitude, where you have quiet and serenity. Your zone contains no electronic devices, no work tools, no hassles, and no scheduling boards. And getting carried into a thought stream of worry, rumination, and pressure is off-limits in this special place.

You could have a special room for meditation, prayer, or contemplation. If you don't have a room, find an area with minimum traffic flow. Make an altar containing special mementos and favorite photographs that raise pleasant memories and peaceful feelings. A corner of your den or bedroom where you wear earphones and listen to relaxing music works as a getaway. Or you could try a screened porch where you listen to nature sounds and watch Mother Nature conduct her magic.

Recharging Your Batteries

A great way to recharge your batteries is to turn your bathroom or hot tub into a spa for the day. Place scented candles around the tub, play soft music in the background, and draw a warm bath with bubble bath, essential oils, or rose petals. Have soft, cotton oversized towels to wrap yourself into once you're finished. Then dim the lights, slide into the tub, sip your favorite beverage, and soak away the stresses of the day.

De-Stress by Accentuating Sensory Comfort

When creating a stress-free environment, think of as many ways as you can to accentuate the five senses. Studies show that pleasant sights, sounds, smells, tastes, and touch act as antidotes to environmental stress and lower your stress level. This section contains ways to transform your home into a stress-free, calming place, where you can kick off your shoes and unwind from pressures of the day. The main quality of a stress-free atmosphere is one that appeals to your five senses in a completely different way from the sensory experience you associate with daily pressures.

Your Stress-Proof Haven

To create a stress-proof haven, neutralize your surroundings from the loud noises, harsh sights, rough textures, offensive odors, and strong tastes of your stressful world. You can use the following guidelines to create greater sensory comfort in your personal space:

> ➤ Listen to quiet sounds such as soft music or nature sounds
>
> ➤ Dim the lights and decorate the space with relaxing colors like blue, green, and yellow
>
> ➤ Use soothing textures such as cushioned slippers, cozy blankets, or a comfy velvety throw
>
> ➤ Introduce calming smells such as scented candles or simmering potpourri to your space
>
> ➤ Eat comfort food such as a warm bowl of soup or a steaming cup of herbal tea

Truth Serum

Researchers at the University of Miami found that guided imagery and music decrease cortisol levels, fatigue, and mood disturbance. Other studies show that a musical refuge can bring you down from an adrenaline high and increase serotonin levels in your brain. Soft music lowers heart rate and blood pressure and helps you sleep better and longer. A delicate blend of music combined with soothing nature sounds—such as waterfalls, raindrops, a rushing brook, or ocean waves—activates the calming parts of your brain and helps you relax. My favorite nature CDs are *Songbirds of Spring*, *Babbling Brook*, *Tropical Jungle*, and my all-time favorite, *Frog Talk*.

Stress Vocab

Aromatherapy is a form of alternative medicine that uses natural oils and other aromatic compounds extracted from flowers, bark, stems, leaves, and roots to improve mood and mental and physical well-being.

Aromatherapy: Nothing Fishy About It

Aromatherapy is gaining attention as an alternative treatment for stress, infections, and other health problems. The practice is widely believed to calm your mind and help you physically heal.

Olfactory Comfort Healing

Many people claim that inhaled aromas from essential oils have positive effects on your brain by stimulating the limbic system through the olfactory system. When massaged into your skin, oils travel through the bloodstream to relieve pain, enhance mood, and improve mental functioning. There are also claims that aromatherapy reduces your risk of contracting colds and flu. Here are some other claims:

➤ Lavender has healing properties when applied to skin burns and puts you at ease.

➤ Lemon oil relaxes, lifts your mood, and acts as a stress antidote.

➤ Jasmine aromas have an uplifting effect on your mind and fight depression.

➤ Chamomile and geranium have a calming effect and aid in stress relief.

Uplifting Your Mood Makes Scents

Certain scents are said to evoke pleasant memories of the past that can have a soothing effect on you. You can find scented candles with alluring smells for all four seasons:

➤ A vanilla-spice candle fills a winter room with warmth.

➤ A blue agave and cacao candle from desert flowers carries undertones of lime, grapefruit, and cinnamon, hinting of spring.

➤ A chilled sangria candle fills a room with the scent reminiscent of lazy summer days.

➤ A French bourbon vanilla is an autumn-like candle with scents of sweet bourbon.

Recharging Your Batteries

The jury is still out on the scientific benefits of aromatherapy. But many people swear by it, saying that certain aromas calm them down. And I'm a believer. During winter months at my house, we keep a simmering pot of potpourri on the kitchen stove. The scent of fresh cinnamon, clove, and ginger root permeates the house, triggering happy memories from the past and lifting our spirits during the gray, cold days.

And research supports these claims. One study found that flooding your room with pleasant smells like scented candles or fresh flowers promotes pleasant dreams while bad odors trigger nightmares. So what do you have to lose? Get the litter box out of your room and put a bouquet of gardenias by your bed. Sweet dreams.

Color Yourself Calm

Did you know that you can color yourself calm? Believe it or not, you can actually use color as a stress management tool when you choose room colors that calm and relax you. Studies show that colors affect your emotional state, raising or lowering your stress level.

Red excites and stimulates you and makes your heart beat faster, whereas more natural tones of green (think trees and grass) and blue (think sky and ocean) have calming effects that relax you. Yellow (think sunlight and daffodils) is the feel-good color. And scientists have found that in yellow rooms you're likely to feel cheerful because yellow triggers the release of serotonin, the feel-good chemical in your brain.

Visual Rest: The Eyes Have It

Another way to provide visual comfort is to place inspirational books on positive thinking, meditation, massage, yoga, or spirituality around the room. Not only do they have visual appeal, but they are handy if you want to flip through them or read a passage or two daily. A few of my favorites are *Stillness Speaks* by Eckhart Tolle, *Quiet Mind: One-Minute Retreats from a Busy World* by David Kundtz, and *Journey to the Heart: Daily Meditations on the Path to Freeing Your Soul* by Melody Beattie.

Your space should also have reminders of trips you've taken and good times you've shared with special people. You can enhance visual comfort by decorating your personal space with items that evoke pleasant memories and feelings such as souvenirs and photos of celebrations and gatherings with friends and loved ones. You can also doll up your surroundings with collections and purchases that have sentimental value such as carvings, paintings, pottery, and textured wall hangings.

Breathe Natural Life into Your Personal Space

Another way to create a calm and relaxing environment is to bring in as much of the natural world as you can. By capitalizing on natural sights and sounds, you bring the outdoors inside. This section contains some ways to breathe natural life into your personal space.

Views of Nature

Studies show that a view of nature from your window reduces stress. Capitalize on scenes of wooded areas, water, sunsets, landscapes, or wildlife. Bring as much outside indoors as possible by arranging your living areas facing the views. If you don't have a view, nature photos or paintings will do. An opened window with a soft breeze and nature sounds add a natural touch. Or consider a tabletop waterfall that makes calming babbling sounds as the water flows over small pebbles.

Recharging Your Batteries

Studies show that artificial lighting such as fluorescent lights increases cortisol stress hormone levels. But you can turn your house into a stress-free zone with natural lighting, which is more restful and lowers stress levels.

So make sure you capture as much natural sunlight as you can. Keep your blinds or shutters open to create a sunny atmosphere. Remove window treatments, furniture, or objects that block daylight. Wash the inside and outside of windows regularly. If all else fails, studies show that full-spectrum lights give you the benefits of natural lighting and elevate your mood if you have seasonal affective disorder (SAD).

Plants and Flowers

If you live in an urban area or a place where there's not much Mother Nature to harness, bring in green plants, fresh flowers, or create a terrarium. I used to live in a city loft with views of buildings and asphalt. But my high ceilings and wide spaces accommodated huge trees that breathed natural life into the loft, warming what otherwise would have been a cold atmosphere. No matter the size of your living space, there's always room for a potted plant or window box of blooming flowers.

Animals and Pets

You can add a touch of Mother Nature with an aquarium or fish bowl full of freshwater or saltwater fish. And stroking a pet whether it's a bird, cat, or dog lowers your blood pressure and relaxes you, which is especially welcome after a hard day.

My philosophy has always been to bring as much of nature into my living space as possible because of its restorative properties. In addition to my yellow-naped Amazon parrot, I live with four dogs and a terrarium of tropical plants. I also have raccoons, bears, and assorted wildlife on my deck daily. But I suggest leaving your wildlife friends outside and admiring them from afar.

Discover Your Inner Sanctuary

Deep within you is a stillness to which you can retreat and gain insight and peace. There, you'll find an inward quietness—a resource to help you navigate through stressful days. During these soothing moments, you gain clarity and find answers to daily pressures.

You can create this special place of calm and harmony anytime, anywhere you can be alone: meditating, praying, watching nature, practicing yoga, or just sitting quietly and contemplating life.

The Doctor Of Calm Is In

Within you there is a stillness and a sanctuary to which you can retreat at any time and be yourself.

—Herman Hesse

When you take reflective moments out of each day to spend with yourself, stress doesn't seem so overwhelming nor life so unmanageable. My prescription: Create your own retreat center, where you can take time out of the rat race. Begin quieting your mind with an initial once-daily dose of a still activity for five minutes. Then, slowly increase the frequency and length of time until stillness becomes a building block to your well-being and to being well. Here's to outsmarting your stress!

CHAPTER 18

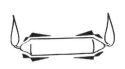

Sidestepping Work Stress and Job Burnout

In This Chapter

- ➤ Types of work stress
- ➤ Discovering your job stressors
- ➤ Stressful workplaces
- ➤ Dealing with job loss and job uncertainty

In this chapter, you'll discover that most people's jobs are their biggest sources of stress and that everybody has some degree of job stress. You'll find out how stressful your job is and how you can manage it. Plus, you'll learn healthy ways to handle unreasonable job demands, job uncertainty, and job loss.

Out with 9 to 5 and In with 24/7

"Workin' nine to five," Dolly Parton sang, "It's enough to drive you / crazy if you let it." And she's right. It will, *if you let it*. But you don't have to worry about 9 to 5 workdays anymore. In the twenty-first century, we have the 24/7 workdays and the technologically driven work culture with soaring job pressures. "It's enough to drive you crazy if you let it." The key is not to let it, but that's easier said than done.

Janet is a case in point. A victim of downsizing, she has gone from a $70,000 a year paycheck to scrambling for work. At a time when she thought she'd be scaling the corporate ladder, bills have stacked up and she has plummeted into a deep depression.

Stress Vocab

Work stress is the pressure you feel when job demands—such as hours or responsibilities—outweigh your ability to manage them.

Work Pressures Can Make You Sick

A 2000 Gallup Poll reported that 80 percent of American workers suffer some type of work stress. And half say they need help learning how to manage it. Some work stress is normal. But as you see with Janet, after an extreme wallop, job stress can leave you with a whiplash, harming your health and interfering with your ability to function.

Research shows that work stress creates all kinds of illnesses. Constant job pressures keep your defenses on high alert, raising your risk of high blood pressure, type 2 diabetes, chronic pain, and a lowered immune system. Studies show that job-related illness has become a worldwide problem.

Trending Now from the Smart Files

Here are some statistics on worldwide job illness:

➤ Studies of American workers show that 60 percent of women say stress is their number one problem on the job and that women are at risk of heart disease linked to work stress.

➤ In the Netherlands, surveys show that leisure illness—which occurs when workers get sick after taking time off and trying to relax on weekends and vacations—affects 3 percent of the work force.

➤ In the United States, the National Occupational Health and Safety Commission reports that work-related stress accounts for the longest stretches of absenteeism.

➤ In Japan, an estimated 5 percent of strokes and heart attacks are due to what the Japanese call *karoshi*-death, death from overwork.

Identifying Your Job Stressors

There are many types of on-the-job stressors that can challenge you, ranging anywhere from trouble with arranging day care to poor pay. Stress is different from person to person, and sometimes work stressors that burden you become another person's challenge and vice versa. Whether or not you are weighed down depends on the nature of your job and your psychological makeup, work habits, and overall general health.

What stresses you out at work? Circle your job stressors from the list below. If you have others, jot them in your stress journal along with the ones you've circled here.

➤ Heavy workload

➤ Poor working conditions

➤ Long hours

➤ Worry over budget cuts and layoffs

➤ Unreasonable company expectations

➤ Competition for promotions

➤ Commuting problems

➤ Performance pressures

➤ Trapped in a miserable job

➤ Lack of career challenge

➤ Employees work at cross-purposes

➤ Dread of facing a negative coworker, demanding client, or the boss from hell

Recharging Your Batteries

Are you a desk potato? Research shows that 80 percent of US jobs are sedentary. But your body isn't designed to be deskbound for long periods of time. Prolonged sitting reduces blood and oxygen flow, causes weight gain, and leads to heart disease and type 2 diabetes, so it's important to take frequent work breaks.

Consider taking short five-minute strolls outside on a nice day or up and down a flight of stairs in bad weather. Or exercise at your desk. Stand up, breathe deeply, shake, twist, and stretch out the built-up tension. Take a few seconds to reach high. Let yourself feel the stretch as you elongate your body and notice where tension is held and released. Shake the part of your body where you sense tension. As you continue to stretch, bring your attention to each part of your body that has remained tight. Bend over and touch your toes and feel that stretch, letting the tension in your body evaporate.

Overtime Hours and Work Stress

Long workweeks in high-pressured jobs contribute to the risk of burnout and heart attack. British researchers found that workers who put in more than eleven hours a day were 67 percent more likely to have a heart attack, compared to those who put in fewer hours. Plus, employees working double or triple duty, carrying heavier workloads to make up for job cuts, are the most likely to be plagued by stress-induced headaches, muscle pain, metabolic disorders, and fatigue outside the workplace. Other research shows that highly effective managers work an average of fifty-two hours a week, compared to less productive managers who average seventy hours. Managers who work longer hours also suffer greater anxiety, depression, burnout, and twice the number of health-related problems than managers putting in fewer hours.

Stress Vocab

Job Burnout is the physical and emotional exhaustion created by prolonged work stress. It can show up as depression, anxiety, despair, fatigue, a negative job attitude, and loss of interest in work.

Physical and Behavioral Signs of Job Stress

Studies show that chronic work stress can be just as bad for your mental and physical well-being as smoking and lack of exercise. Prolonged work stress can lead to job burnout. According to a 2011 CareerBuilder survey, 45 percent of American workers complain that their workload is too heavy and 77 percent say they have job burnout.

What about you? Are you a member of the burned-out generation? Are you a restless grump with coworkers? Do you feel overwhelmed by a swirling work fog? These are just some of the warning signs of job stress. From the list below, notice if the signs of work stress hit home. Check off the ones that apply to you.

Here are some physical signs of work stress:

➤ Headaches

➤ Fatigue

➤ Gastrointestinal problems

➤ Muscle pains

➤ Chest pains

> ➤ Shortness of breath

> ➤ Nervous tics

> ➤ Compromised immune system

> ➤ Frequent illnesses

> ➤ Insomnia or restlessness

> ➤ High blood pressure

Here are some behavioral signs of work stress:

> ➤ Inconsistent work quality

> ➤ Drop in productivity

> ➤ Difficulty concentrating on tasks

> ➤ Increased mistakes and errors in judgment

> ➤ Inability to fulfill responsibilities

> ➤ Outbursts of temper and argumentativeness

> ➤ Irritability and impatience

> ➤ Job boredom

> ➤ Trouble getting to work on time

> ➤ Chronic absenteeism

> ➤ Accident prone

Truth Serum

For crying out loud! Research shows that a noisy workplace can cause stress hormones to rise to unhealthy levels—a condition that constricts coronary arteries and reduces blood supply to the heart. One study found that people exposed to chronic loud noise on the job were twice as likely to have heart disease and heart attacks as those who toiled in quieter places.

Is It Your Job or Your Work Style?

A 2006 global survey by *World Business* revealed that 49 percent of workers said overwork is encouraged by their company. And a CareerBuilder survey shows that 49 percent of employers expect workers to check in with the office while they're away.

In one bank, an executive said top managers lead with, "We expect you to change tires going 80 miles an hour." He said employees constantly check their BlackBerrys and Androids during meetings, at lunch, and on the way to the restroom. To survive in that stressful work culture, employees say they can't afford to focus on just one thing at a time. Multitasking is their essential lifeboat to keep from drowning in a sea of work.

On the flip side, some employees are attracted to high-stress careers. They pressure themselves with unrealistic job demands, fail to monitor work habits, and allow their careers to trump other aspects of their lives. For instance, the CEO who sneaks a cell phone and laptop into the hospital room after she has just undergone major surgery or the attorney who cannot say no, schedules clients around the clock, and burns himself out.

Are You Married to the Job?

Are you the type of worker who dreams about being in the office while on the ski slopes, an employee who works more than forty to fifty hours a week, skipping lunch breaks to eat at your desk, staying in constant contact with the office on weekends, holidays, and vacations, feeling nervous or antsy when away from work? If so, you could be among the ranks of those who consider workaholism to be the new cocaine, using your job to escape from personal problems and creating more stress in your life than you're aware of. Take the Risky Business test in Appendix A to see if any of the workaholic warning signs apply to you.

Warning Signs of a Stressful Workplace

Some businesses try to get a greater bang for their buck. They want to make sure that every dollar spent contributes to the company's growth, sacrificing people for profit. Many companies operate from the top to bottom through a structure that strips management layers in order to remain competitive, employing four people to do the work of five. Power picnics are replacing company picnics that were once a family affair so that companies can squeeze in more work during the annual event. And power lunches are replacing office lunch breaks.

Excessive corporate demand combined with wireless technology risks company exploitation of workers who feel they must be available 24/7. Some organizations set tight, impossible deadlines, hint at nonexistent competitors, and tell employees that clients are dissatisfied even when they are not. These corporate tactics create paranoia, stress, and a prolonged adrenaline rush among the workforce; employees never know for sure which crises are real and which are fabrications. Could your company be one of these?

Is Your Job Hazardous to Your Health?

Does your workplace put profit before your well-being, promoting stress and burnout, or are you fortunate enough to work for a company that considers human factors and nurtures its employees? To see if you toil in a toxic work site, grade your job by taking the test in Appendix A called Is Your Job Hazardous to Your Health?

Shock Absorber

No one can tell you to quit your job without knowing the intimate details of your work and personal life. That's your call. But if it's all you can find, even if you're not thrilled with it, you don't want to trade one problem for another by being unemployed. And if your job is tolerable and pays the bills, you have to weigh the financial advantages in light of your job's negative aspects, plus the other factors in your life such as the people who are dependent on you, amount of debt, and so on. So if you're debating whether to quit or stay put, before you throw in the towel make sure your emotions don't bias your decision. And think it through thoroughly.

Work Habits That Can Stress You Out

Not all stress can be blamed on the workplace. Sometimes stress can be caused by your style of approaching tasks. Here are ten work habits that can lead to stress:

➤ Focusing on the external world of doing with little attention to your internal world of being.

➤ Quantifying what you do (seeing it and measuring it) in order to feel good about yourself

➤ Putting your self-care needs last until all the work is done

➤ Having difficulty being in the present moment

➤ Focusing too much on the final product instead of on the progress you're making

➤ Scheduling yourself to the hilt, allowing for little or no flexibility or spontaneity

➤ Defining yourself and others by accomplishments instead of human qualities

➤ Feeling incomplete and unfinished without something to keep you busy

➤ Engaging in self-criticism so that you never seem to accomplish enough

➤ Taking work too seriously instead of lightening up

Jot down personal habits from this list and any others that might contribute to your work stress such as people pleasing, impatience, procrastination, or perfectionism.

Rebooting Your Work Health

There are always aspects of job stress that you won't be able to eliminate. But within limits, there are parts of it that you can manage. The solution? Pay attention to exactly what stresses you out at work—it can be an eye-opener. Then take steps to reduce your stress and boost your health.

Devising a Work Health Plan

It's usually not the entire job that causes stress but one or two aspects of it. Now that you've had some food for thought, look over your two earlier lists: workplace stressors and personal work habits. What do you come up with? Does your stress come from work site demands, your personal work style, or a combination? From the information you've gleaned, note how much comes from you and how much comes from your workplace. Put a check mark beside the ones you can change. In your journal, note what changes you need to make to become a better manager of job stress so you don't burn out. And then take action.

Shock Absorber

For health's sake, make sure you realize you've hit your breaking point long before stress warning signs set in. Instead of pushing past them, cushion your workday to soften stress blows. Refrain from putting yourself under unrealistic deadlines. Replace deadlines with "lifelines" by spreading job tasks over reasonable time frames. And build time cushions between appointments. When you're running late, it adds to your stress level. Try leaving for work ten or fifteen minutes earlier so you won't start your day in a hurry. Ease into your workday instead of catapulting into it. And unplug at the end of the day. You'll be more efficient the next morning when you protect your time off.

Tips on Coming Up for Air

Like most people, you're probably not aware that your stress response is on high alert when you're working. You get swept up in the day-to-day minutiae and don't realize the toll—both physical and mental—job stress is taking on you. But even seemingly innocuous work sites, including home offices, can pose health risks. Here are tips to reboot your health when you feel like you're crashing from job pressures:

➤ Be mindful of your surroundings: Paying attention to what's around you reduces stress and generates more performance energy in a demanding job. Take off your socks and shoes and feel your toes against the floor. Pay close attention to how the floor feels against your feet: cold, warm, soft, hard? If you have an opened window, focus on the sounds of chirping birds or inhale the fragrance of a flower.

➤ Change your scenery: Getting outside even if it's only for twenty minutes, not only gives your fatigued mind a break, but also boosts your mood. Dine away from your desk or take a walk around the block or in a park.

➤ Give your workstation a makeover: A disorganized or sloppy work area can raise tensions. Does your desk look like a tsunami struck? If so, a tidy work space can reduce stress and establish feelings of calm and control.

➤ Dial back on overtime: To cut your health risks, reduce overtime work when possible. Toil by the adage of working smarter, not longer.

➤ Meditate: Meditating or contemplating at your desk for just five minutes is restorative. It helps you unwind, clear your head, and refresh your mind, body, and spirit.

➤ Stay fit outside the office: Think of your work site as the Olympics. Your physical and mental endurance at work hinges on being in good shape. Prepare yourself for your workdays by taking care of your physical health outside of work. Prime yourself with good nutrition, vigorous exercise, and ample sleep. Avoid nicotine and use alcohol in moderation.

Saying No Instead of Yo to Unreasonable Job Demands

Everybody has a breaking point. Learn to be a better stress manager when you're tired or burned out. Listen to your body for stress signals; take care of yourself with breaks when those signals go off. But what if you discover that the majority of your stress comes from your workplace? You can't fire your boss. You can't take over the company and restructure it, but you can take a number of actions.

Set Boundaries with Work

Don't let job stress metastasize into your personal time. Limit the use of wireless devices during private hours and enjoy relationships, hobbies, and other areas of life outside work. You'll have more balance, higher energy, a clearer head, and fewer health problems on the job.

Prioritize and Delegate Your Workload

Some job tasks are more important than others, so learn to decide what must come first. Have your priorities clear and practical. The clearer you are on what you want to accomplish and how you plan to accomplish it, the more focused and efficient and less stressed you'll be. Decide which aspects of your job are key, and focus first on the things that require immediate attention. Put nonessentials on the back burner or farm them out to an assistant or coworker.

Learn to ask others for help when you need it. If you're the type who has trouble turning a project over to someone else, remember that delegating helps you perform optimally. Review your workload and decide what part you can give to an assistant, intern, or coworker. When you share the load, you'll have more energy, and you'll feel more like a team player—and so will your coworkers.

Evaluate Your Company's Demands

Don't wait for your company to decide what's best for you.

No matter how dedicated you are, evaluate your job and overall life to decide what's reasonable for you. Decide how far you're willing to go to meet company demands. Be prepared to put your foot down when you believe your employer oversteps those bounds. There are many occasions on the job when you have a choice to stay late or work weekends. You may be reluctant to say no, but drawing the line without guilt when overloaded is a healthy thing to do for yourself.

Schedule a Meeting with Your Boss

If you discover your workload is out of line, use your situation as a talking point when you meet with your manager. Ask if there's another way to divide up job tasks. When deadlines are too tight, negotiate them with your supervisor. Deadlines can almost always be modified. Develop a plan explaining the need for an extension, and suggest a revised time frame. Align your goals with those of the company, and work with your manager to prioritize projects.

Ask about company expectations and find out exactly what performance goals you must meet to receive an excellent review rating. Experts say that 99 percent of the time work hours are not a big factor in performance reviews. This action ensures that you won't be downgraded for not putting in extra hours. Without complaining, talk over your concerns with your employer. Make sure your boss understands your point of view, the importance of your personal life, and your expectations concerning job demands.

Reach Out to Coworkers for Support

More companies are realizing that work stress is a major health and safety issue and that it is to their advantage to have healthy employees. Big corporations like General Mills are insisting that employees take their vacation time. Other companies are finding unique ways to support employees and de-stress work environments: paid paternity leave, job sharing, flextime, onsite stress-reduction classes.

Studies show that workers with low social support on the job were twice as likely to die over a twenty-year period than people with supportive coworkers. If you feel like your workload is unsustainable and unfair, reach out to coworkers to see if they're working the same long hours and ask how they're managing it. If colleagues are also stressed, establish support group meetings before or after work to deal with job stress. When appropriate, enlist your boss as a resource, including him or her in group meetings to find constructive solutions to stress-related problems.

Truth Serum

Organizational research shows that optimists achieve more career success than pessimists. Sometimes offices become dumping grounds for grouser negativity. Whiners tend to avoid responsibility, beleaguer problems, and expect coworkers to solve problems instead of finding creative solutions themselves. Chronic bellyaching infects workplace morale and sabotages productivity.

Compared to their sunnier coworkers, disgruntled workers have trouble looking on the bright side, working as team players, thinking outside the box, and finding solutions in problems. Coworkers and managers lack confidence in them and don't trust them to lead. Pessimists are shut out of top assignments and suffer derailed careers because they get mired in work stress instead of surmounting it.

Check Your Disgruntled Attitude

Pay close attention to the attitude you bring to the office each day and keep it in check from time to time. Try looking on the bright side and thinking of yourself as a winner instead of a loser. Remind yourself of past challenges that you overcame and of positive comments people made about your previous job performance. Even if your job is stressful, find one or two positive things that you enjoy and look forward to. Hang out with optimistic coworkers instead of negative people who pull you down. Give yourself pep talks as you would give a best friend. Tell yourself, "I can overcome anything I set my mind to." Above all, never give up.

Job Loss and Unemployment Woes

In 2011, the unemployment rate among college-degreed workers shot to its highest level since the U.S. Bureau of Labor Statistics began tracking it in 1970. There is no greater life stressor than the troubling uncertainties brought on by job loss, unemployment, or underemployment. The worries that come with job layoffs, shrinking financial resources, and a questionable job future are enough to make you want to pull your hair out. Financial questions such as how you're going to find a decent-paying job, will you lose your house, how will you get the kids through college, or will you ever be able to retire can even make you sick.

Worried Sick Over Job Uncertainty

Studies show that job loss can lower your immune system, making you more vulnerable to viruses. Workers living with unemployment and underemployment are five times more likely to catch colds than workers without job threats. Job insecurities make you more vulnerable to diseases and worsen existing chronic ailments such as heart disease, diabetes, or depression.

Scientists say that employees living with job uncertainty have worse overall health and more depression than employees who actually lose their jobs. Not knowing is the stressful part.

Truth Serum

William Gallo, a Yale University researcher, found that older adults (fifty years of age and older) who lose their jobs fare worse than the younger unemployed. They have more depression and their risk of heart attack and stroke more than doubles compared to employees who do not lose their jobs.

How to Alleviate Job Insecurities

Many people seek comfort from job insecurity in overeating, alcohol, or smoking —health hazards that only further contribute to physical and emotional illnesses. Studies show that stress over fear of losing a job takes a greater toll on health than actually losing a job. Your best defense against job uncertainty is to manage work stress and make yourself indispensable at work. Here are tips for attending to the basics:

➤ Address stress signals early: Keep yourself fit by getting the sleep, exercise, and balanced diet that your body needs. Avoid junk food, excessive alcohol, and nicotine. These negative behaviors may seem to reduce your anxiety in the short term, but they actually increase your stress level over the long haul.

➤ No matter how bad your hardship, find small escapes that make you happy: Immerse yourself into little things that you can look forward to and that bring you joy: gardening, reading a good novel, having friends over for a potluck dinner, or watching a comedy on TV.

➤ Do something for someone else: Taking your mind off your situation can help you feel better when you take action away from yourself. Research shows that doing for others—especially when you're down and out—creates better emotional health, more inner calm, and a greater sense of self-worth. Take time to visit a sick friend, volunteer for a needy charity, or show a random act of kindness such as letting someone in front of you in the grocery line.

➤ Do your research: Go to job fairs. Talk with employers and find out what they're looking for. The pool is large and you want to stand out, so improve your interviewing skills. Make sure your résumé is neat and grammatically correct and that you have dotted all of your i's and crossed all of your t's.

➤ Take action: Look up the Department of Labor on the Internet to find websites of companies that are hiring. Once you see what's available, apply online. Add this routine to your weekly schedule and be disciplined about it.

Accepting Job Uncertainty

"Accept job uncertainty?" you might ask. "Are you off your rocker?" At first glance it does seem like a pretty tall order. But when you think about it, many aspects of your job are beyond your control: a coworker's attitude, a grumpy boss, threat of budget cuts, impending layoffs, and worry over not finding employment. Job uncertainty is one of the few things you can count on. Studies prove that your ability to accept job uncertainty has a bigger effect on your health than actually losing your job. It reduces stress and brings you peace of mind. Then you can manage what you can, let the rest go, and send stress packing!

The Doctor Of Calm Is In

If uncertainty is unacceptable to you, it turns into fear. If it is perfectly acceptable, it turns into increased aliveness, alertness, and creativity.

—Eckhart Tolle

When job uncertainty is unacceptable to you, it can set up disappointment, resentment, and stress. Are you able to fully surrender to the unknown and make the best of whatever happens? When you can't control workplace situations, find ways to manage them. The acceptance of job uncertainty is a beginning, but it doesn't happen overnight. You need to take baby steps. You can start practicing right now.

My prescription: See if you can lean in the direction of accepting one bothersome work situation that you have no control over. Then notice if acceptance helps you reduce work stress, attain more peace of mind, and manage what you can. This remedy can be taken before, during, or after work until symptoms subside. Here's to outsmarting your stress!

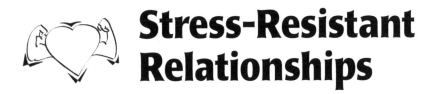

CHAPTER 19

Stress-Resistant Relationships

In this chapter, you'll learn the traits of stress-resistant relationships and get a bird's-eye view of how stress can interfere with good communication. You'll get a chance to examine powerful tools, stress buffers that can prevent or improve stressful relationships. Plus, you'll get tips on the importance of helping others and how over-caring can backfire if you don't have your own house in order.

Making Your Relationships Bloom

Ah, interpersonal relationships. We're affected by them every second of the day—interactions with family members, business associates, neighbors, and the checkout clerk at the local grocery.

When you're consumed by stress, you might feel like shipping your loved ones off to relatives and disappearing into a federal witness protection program. Whether you feel like you can't live with them or you can't live without them, relationships are one of the biggest sources of stress for most people. An American Psychological Association poll shows that 54 percent of Americans say stress causes them to fight with relatives. And one in four says that stress has alienated them from family and friends.

Relationships are not always easy; they usually require time and attention. But the effort you put into them pays off in the long run. Just as your favorite potted plant needs water, fertilizer, and sunlight to bloom, your relationships need tending if they are to thrive. There's a lot you can do to nurture and grow stress-resistant relationships.

Shock Absorber

Are you managing your most important investments? Think of your special relationships as a bank account. Then compare your recent deposits with the withdrawals. As with a bank account, relationships require periodic deposits—time, attention, support, understanding, heart-to-heart talks, encouragement, forgiveness—to stay solvent. These deposits offset withdrawals—demands, stress, criticism, misunderstandings, disagreements, blame—that naturally occur in most relationships.

Consider making a special effort to keep your relationships vital by creating special moments when you try to connect by e-mail, text message, phone, or in the old fashioned way: face-to-face. It's good economics to ask yourself each day what you've deposited into your relationships. Making one daily deposit gives you a stress-proof return on your investment.

Traits of Stress-Resistant Relationships

The key to keeping your relationships vital starts with good communication. Stress-free relationships flow freely and have the following qualities:

➤ Both parties are willing to communicate about problems and concerns.

➤ Neither party is interested in conflict, judging, criticism, or in interpreting each other's actions.

➤ Both parties strive for a harmonious connection through empathy and respect for the other's point of view.

➤ Overwhelming episodes of appreciation are frequent, and both partners are susceptible to receiving love and have an uncontrollable urge to extend it.

Communication Gridlock

Under stress, communication goes down the toilet. Your stress can come out sideways and get displaced on the people you care about the most. But an understanding of how stress erodes interpersonal relationships can help you save, build, or strengthen interpersonal bonds.

Psychologist John Gottman pinpoints four red flags that indicate stress is driving a relationship south and a breakup is imminent:

➤ Criticism

➤ Defensiveness

➤ Withdrawal

➤ Contempt

These four warning signs signal terminal relationship gridlock, usually the result of poor listening and speaking skills.

Are You Stuck in Communication Gridlock?

Gridlock occurs when you're stuck in your own point of view, unwilling to see a problem from another party's vantage point. You communicate your feelings as facts, turning a deaf ear to another person's thoughts and feelings because you've already made up your mind that you're right. And you're determined to force your point of view by commanding, finger pointing, criticizing, and being negative. Gridlock leads to defensiveness, criticism, withdrawal, and contempt from both parties—signs of a complete breakdown of the relationship.

Truth Serum

After breaking up with husband Arnold Schwarzenegger, Maria Shriver said, "It's stressful not knowing what you're doing next." There's a chance you, too, could feel stressed after a breakup, uncertain what the future holds, feeling as if a part of your body has been torn off.

Research shows that a breakup with someone you have affection for can have the same painful feeling in your body as getting burned. It stimulates the same part of the brain that says, "I'm hurt."

Overcoming Gridlock with Effective Communication

You can reduce interpersonal stress and overcome gridlock by learning to communicate well. That means paying attention to how you give and receive information. Using empathy by putting yourself in the other person's situation and temporarily suspending your own viewpoint, for example, sharpens your listening skills. It gives you a clearer understanding of another person's point of view without needing to agree with him or her. Plus, being more mindful of how you respond can give you a sober awareness of how you're perceived by others in relationships. There are actions you can take to remove communication roadblocks.

Avoid Verbal Trespassing

In her book *The Power of Two: Secrets of a Strong and Loving Marriage* Susan Heitler describes a form of communication called verbal trespassing, which can harm relationships. These verbal crossovers are presumptive, heavy-handed, and sound parental. They disregard input about what the other person might be thinking or feeling. If you're like most people, you've probably engaged in one or more crossovers at one time or another without realizing it. Here are five types of verbal trespassing to be aware of with examples of how to avoid them:

> ➤ Mind Reading: You jump to conclusions about what the other person is thinking. You might say something like, "You probably think I'm irresponsible because I lost my cell phone." To sidestep this trespass, check it out: "Do you think I'm irresponsible?"

> ➤ Emotion Reading: You conclude what someone is feeling without evidence. You might say, "You're angry with me because I'm late." To avoid this trespass, ask what the other person is feeling: "Are you angry with me?"

> ➤ Name Calling: You label someone with negative attributes: "You're mean and selfish." To dodge this trespass, step back and speak of yourself, using I messages instead of you messages: "I'm uncomfortable with how we're talking; I'd like to take a time out and come back when we're calmer." When you refer to your own feelings (I messages) instead of pointing your finger (you messages), it reduces defensiveness and tension and promotes more open dialogue.

> ➤ Put Downs: You criticize someone's behavior or habits: "You always pile dirty dishes in the sink instead of putting them in the dishwasher." To reverse this trespass, use, "When you . . . I feel . . ." to communicate how a certain action makes you feel, "When you continue to pile dirty dishes in the sink, it makes me feel like my requests don't matter."

➤ Commanding: You tell someone what to do and expect him or her to do what you say, "Don't eat that; it's bad for you." To prevent this trespass, state your concern or ask a question: "Are you sure you want the meal fried or would you rather have something grilled?"

Listen with Empathy

Now you might be thinking, "But why should I be empathetic to someone who's blasting me, whether loved one or stranger?" That's a good question. Empathetic listening can liberate you from your own narrow and negative thinking, help you see the big picture and refrain from snap judgments. Plugging into someone's point of view can increase understanding and compassion, thereby neutralizing your stress and helping you remain calm. Plus, it raises your ability to connect with someone you care about and neutralizes resentment you might have. You can employ empathetic listening to help settle disputes or keep calm when someone is exploding.

Suppose you've had a pleasant, serene day. Then all of a sudden, someone bounds through the door, cursing, slamming doors, and kicking the dog. Most likely you're upset that he or she is raining on your parade. You might even start slamming things and cursing yourself. But if you know the underlying cause of the rant, your empathetic reaction could buffer your stress.

Suppose the person just got fired, had a wreck, or was just diagnosed with an illness? Whatever the root cause of the unsettling behavior, when you take time to put yourself in someone's place and imagine what it's like for that person, it can mitigate unnecessary turmoil.

Practice Active Listening

Active listening, versus passive listening, actively engages you in what another person is saying and feeling. Your body language moves in sync with the other person's comments and emotions. For example, you might nod your head or lean forward with interest. You have direct eye contact, and you're listening with empathy. You don't give advice unless it's asked for, and you don't hijack the conversation to your point of view or to talk about what you did when the same thing happened to you. You reflect back what the other party says and show support by conveying what you imagine he or she must be feeling. Here's an example of what active listening is and isn't:

Your friend: "The bills are piling up, I still don't have a job, and the stress is getting to me."

What active listening isn't: "That happened to me one time, but I finally got a job. Maybe you need to try harder."

What active listening is: "That's got to be stressful when you don't know where the next paycheck is coming from and you've got bills to pay."

Recharging Your Batteries

One of the best ways to strengthen your intimate relationship is to spend time together. Studies show that talking fifteen minutes a day creates solidarity against outside pressures. And your stressed-out mate has the biggest drop in stress when you're subtly supportive such as by sharing time and attention. Preparing meals jointly and having pleasant mealtime conversations (without the distraction of TV or the Internet) also provide a platform for supportive communication. Another possibility is creating fun pastimes that you share as a couple such as tennis, golf, or walking. Whatever your approach, take a genuine and active interest in your mate's life. Listen to your partner's dreams and disappointments and find out what he or she has been up to and feeling. Research shows that couples who share their daily ups and downs feel happier and more harmonious. Sharing involves your intimate partner in your daily experiences and makes the two of you feel more connected.

Be Assertive

You want to speak your truth in a direct, genuine way. But you also want the other party to hear your concerns. There are ways to achieve both by using assertiveness—that midpoint on the scale between passivity on one end and aggressiveness on the other—to get your point across with strength and clarity.

It's important not to blame others when you feel they make an unreasonable request (it might not seem unreasonable to them) or have not honored a line that you haven't drawn. It's up to you and me to tell others where that line is and when we think they've crossed it. So practice informing the other person calmly and matter-of-factly without making apologies or excuses.

Suppose a friend asks you to help him move on your only Saturday off in a month. You say you'll check your calendar and get back to him (consult yourself first before agreeing to something you're not sure you want to do). After you've given it some thought (about three seconds), you decide you need that day for yourself. You inform your friend in a calm, genuine, matter-of-fact manner with something like, "I'd like to help you out, but that's my only day off in weeks and I've made other plans." And you probably would like to help him out, but you do have other plans: to take care of yourself. When you stand up for yourself with consideration and respect, usually other people will follow your lead.

State Your Frustration as a Desire

Start to see your criticisms and frustrations as desires stated in a negative way. Then turn them inside out and communicate your desire. For example, when you want a procrastinator to stop holding everybody back, replace the critical comment, "You never complete your work on time and you're holding everybody back" with a comment of desire, "I like the efficiency of things running smoother when you meet the deadlines we set." When you want your spouse to keep a cleaner kitchen, say something like, "I appreciate it when you put dirty dishes in the dishwasher" instead of, "How many times have I asked you to stop piling dirty dishes in the sink?"

Use a Positive Approach

Use the Burger King approach, or the bun-meat-bun method of communication. Nobody likes to be blasted with negative comments, but if you ease into them with a genuinely positive statement (the bun), it makes it easier for the recipient to hear your beef. Then you close with another bun (positive statement).

This method of communication allows you to give critical feedback in a way that is honest and direct and that allows others to hear you without getting defensive. It softens your critical comments by sandwiching potentially negative comments between two positives: "This report has a lot of merit. I would change the wording in the last paragraph. But overall you've done a great job."

Effective Communication Through Love Languages

Do you know your love language? Chances are if you're in an intimate relationship, you hit a snag because you and your intimate partner speak different love languages. No matter how hard you try to express yourself in English, if your mate only understands Chinese, your ability to communicate and connect is stalled. So it is with the expression of love. Your love language and that of your mate could be as different as English and Chinese. But when you learn each other's primary love language and speak it, it helps you develop mutual empathy, appreciation, and strong communication.

Stress Vocab

Love Language is the unique way in which you send and receive expressions of love from your intimate partner.

Five Types of Love Languages

In his book *The 5 Love Languages: The Secret to Love That Lasts,* Gary Chapman names five different languages of love:

➤ Words of Affirmation: You communicate appreciation, encouragement, kindness, humility, and empathy, seeing the world from your intimate partner's point of view.

➤ Quality Time: You spend time together, giving your full attention to your spouse or partner, have meaningful conversations in which you share your deepest feelings and experiences, or enjoy activities in which you both share an interest.

➤ Receiving Gifts: You give and accept money or gifts that represent an expression of love, or you gift yourself by being emotionally present during your mate's time of need.

➤ Acts of Service: You perform an action that you know would please your partner such as cooking a favorite meal, washing the car, or doing the grocery shopping.

➤ Physical Touch: You are physically intimate in the form of hugging, kissing, holding hands, giving back rubs, or having sexual intercourse.

Truth Serum

Physical touch is a powerful way to communicate caring and kindness without saying a word. Scientists say that a gentle touch when you're communicating with someone—even when asking a stranger for directions—elicits more support from the other person. Being touched is calming, and it releases oxytocin, creating safety and trust and establishing a platform for settling differences. So if you're comfortable with touching, go ahead—snuggle, hold hands, hug, or give a back rub; it bonds your relationship.

Quiz: What is Your Love Language?

Answering the following questions can give you a clue to your (or your partner's) love language and a clearer picture of how you receive your mate's love:

➤ What does your intimate partner do or fail to do that frustrates you the most or hurts you deeply? (The opposite of what hurts you or frustrates you could indicate your love language.)

➤ What do you need emotionally from your spouse or partner that you don't get enough of? (Your unmet emotional needs are likely indicators of what would make you feel loved.)

➤ How do you usually show love to your mate? (Because we tend to love our intimate partners in ways we would like to be loved, your way of expressing love is often a clue to what would also make you feel loved.)

➤ What is your idea of an ideal spouse or partner?

Answers to these questions can give you a picture of your love language and that of your partner. The next step is to share your discovery and then practice speaking each other's love languages on a regular basis.

Shock Absorber

You've heard it said time and again that opposites attract. And it's true. In most intimate relationships, one party is a *rock* and one is a *bird*. Rocks play their cards close to their vests, keep their feet firmly planted on the ground, are organized and logical, and usually have things under control. Birds show their cards. They could care less about order and organization. They are open, playful, spontaneous, flexible, and flow with the moment. They are often more creative and intuitive than rocks.

These differences can be sources of major conflict. But they don't have to be. One style is not more right or wrong. Actually, the rock and bird are a union made in heaven. The rock provides stability and the bird provides levity—both necessary ingredients for a balanced match.

Think about who's the rock and who's the bird in your relationship. Then see if you can discover the value in your partner's style. Once you start to look at the differences as a plus instead of a minus, you'll inject less stress and more harmony in your relationship.

Your Past Relationships are Still Present

One of the things that makes Mark sizzle is when people let him down or don't follow through on what they say. When his wife would forget to mail a letter or make a phone call for him, Mark went ballistic. His extreme reaction was out of proportion to the incident. What he eventually learned by paying attention to his outbursts was that when someone let him down in a big or small way, his amygdala (see Chapter 9) flooded his current new emotional experiences with a past emotional memory, causing him to overreact. In a split second, the library in his brain held the memory of his boyhood disappointments and the broken promises by his alcoholic father. He learned as a boy that he couldn't depend on adults to do what they said. And he continued to reexperience in his marriage the belief that grown-ups are unreliable.

Stress Vocab

Imago is the unconscious blueprint you carry from childhood that guides the kind of mate you'll be attracted to in your adult intimate relationships.

Romantic Attraction

Situations in the present that are similar to those that have been recorded by the reptilian, or old, brain trigger the amygdala, which kicks into survival mode. The science behind romantic attraction shows that your brain tries to recreate the conditions of your upbringing (good or bad) in order to correct them.

In his famous book *Getting the Love You Want: A Guide for Couples*, Harville Hendrix explains romantic attraction in terms of what he calls the imago (pronounced eh-MAH-go, Latin for "image").

The imago works such that your romantic attraction is based on a composite picture of the caretakers who influenced you most strongly at an early age. When an imago match is made deep in your brain, a surge of interest in the other person occurs. You and your intimate partner activate in each other stressors that plunge you back into the central conflicts of your upbringing in order to have it turn out better the second time around.

Truth Serum

If you're like most people, you were swept off your feet when you first met the love of our life. You swooned. Your heart leaped. And your partner's virtues naturally stood out from the vices. Then after a few years into the relationship, you started to see the flip side of the coin: all the things that bug you. People say things like, "Boy, has she changed!" or "He's not the same man I married." But the truth is that she hasn't changed, and, yes, he's *exactly* the same man you married. Psychologists say you're just seeing the other side.

The things that cause problems in intimate relationships are the flip side of the things that originally attracted you. Think about it this way: virtues contain vices, strength contains willfulness, stability contains control, spontaneity contains abandon. In intimate relationships, you get a package deal.

A Match Made in Heaven?

Without realizing it, you click with a mate who in some way matches your imago template. You surround yourself with people and situations that feel comfortable and familiar—even when you vow to avoid harmful situations, you end up in them anyhow, fully knowing the consequences of your actions. You go back to the same types of people for the same rejections and keep trying to solve problems in the same old ways that don't work. And if you're like the average person, you say something like, "I'll never hook up with an ogre like my father." But, no matter what your conscious intentions, you are attracted to someone who has your caretakers' positive and negative traits, and, typically, the negative traits are more influential.

Returning to the Scene of the Crime

You're basically looking for a mate who duplicates your parents' inadequacies. Your old brain is returning to the scene of the crime, so to speak, to right the wrongs of your childhood. You expect your partner to make up for the problem but the unfortunate consequence is that, because of the imago match, you get re-wounded.

To change your pattern of attraction, you'll have to figure out what's not working and change it instead of repeating it. The first step is to pay attention to the red flags and recognize what's happening inside of you when you're attracted to someone.

For example, suppose in hindsight you realize you keep getting stuck in relationships with emotionally distant partners. That could be your imago at work, which means your blueprint probably came from emotionally absent caretakers. Your imago is trying to fill that void with the only kind of relationship you've ever known: emotionally unavailable people.

So next time you fly off the handle, see if you can relate it to a pattern of feelings you've had before. The key is to recognize your triggers—the stored information in your old brain that keeps coming up for you. If you're honest, you'll start to see a pattern of when you're angry, sad, hurt, or scared. And you'll see it's an inner reaction that causes you to sizzle, not the present person or circumstance. Once you can separate your inner library from the present upsetting situation, you can make a more mature, rational response that makes you more stress resistant.

Antistress Advantages of Helping Others

Helping others through good deeds actually can reduce your stress. The obvious benefit is that you get a break from your own stressful burdens. When you reach out to help someone else, you forget about your worries for a while. But that's just for starters. Contributing, giving, volunteering, donating, and performing kind acts, no matter how small or brief, connect you to other people (and animals) in a deeply meaningful, humane way.

Reaching out to others can make your life feel worthwhile and give you a sense of purpose, meaning, and self-worth. And, depending on the type of giving, you get greater appreciation for your life compared to the less fortunate people you're serving. If those benefits aren't convincing enough, consider the scientific fact that volunteers who regularly care for others have more vitality, better health, and longer lives than people who don't volunteer. Now are you sold on the idea that it's better to give than to receive?

Recharging Your Batteries

It might sound odd to you, but helping others has a boomerang effect. Commonly know as the helper's high, performing good deeds boosts your mood, calms you down, and relieves you of stress-related illnesses. The bursts of euphoria come from dopamine and endorphin squirts released in your brain. Plus, tending and befriending (as was mentioned in Chapter 9) swells your oxytocin level, softening stress's potent punch.

Medical studies show that the saliva of compassionate people contains more immunoglobulin A, which is an antibody that fights off infection. In addition to boosting the immune system, brain scans of benevolent people show that generosity gave them a calmer disposition, less stress, better emotional health, and higher self-worth.

What Are You Waiting for?

So what are you waiting for? Perform an act of kindness today, whether it's running an errand for a friend, taking friendship trays to shut-ins, letting a harried shopper in front of you in line, or making a contribution to your favorite charity. The formula is to match your time constraints, resources, natural talents, skills, and interests with one or more needs in your community. There are more avenues for generosity than space permits on this page. But here are a few examples to trigger your creative juices:

➤ Tutor children in math or reading after school

➤ Assist patients in hospice or in a hospital

➤ Usher at community theater productions

➤ Volunteer at an animal shelter or humane society

- ➤ Sponsor a disadvantaged child or family in another culture or take a mission trip to another country
- ➤ Lead a 12-Step meeting or Sunday school class
- ➤ Participate in a walkathon to raise money for breast cancer, HIV, or another important cause
- ➤ Work for a homeless shelter or Habitat for Humanity
- ➤ Answer an emergency hotline
- ➤ Advocate as a guardian *ad litem* for abused and neglected children
- ➤ Serve on the board of a local agency
- ➤ Volunteer for the Red Cross or Salvation Army
- ➤ Donate old clothes, appliances, or furniture to Goodwill

Can You Care Too Much?

"It's a quarter after one, I'm all alone and I need you now," Lady Antebellum sings. "And I don't know how I can do without, I just need you now." These beautiful lyrics illustrate how the desperation of needing someone can lead to codependent or careaholic relationships. The word *careaholic* might sound odd. And you might even ask, "How can you care too much?" But there's a difference between healthy caring and careaholism.

Caring Versus Careaholism

Careaholics overload themselves with other people's problems as a distraction from their own worries and stresses. Caring is counterproductive when helping others becomes a means to avoid or self-medicate your own pain. This is sometimes called codependency. If you're focused on taking care of someone else, you don't have to think about your own burdens. And if you have unfinished business of your own, you're not likely to let someone else struggle with theirs.

But the inability of careaholics to focus on themselves eventually works against them. Their inability to say no and the tendency to put themselves last takes its toll. When careaholics don't have anyone needing them, they start to feel empty and lacking in purpose. As the stress cycle kicks in, the relief (over-caring) eventually becomes the problem.

Careaholics hit bottom when they reach compassion burnout (see Chapter 4), which shows up in a variety of ways: fatigue, gastrointestinal irritations, insomnia, despair, hypertension, or depression.

Stress Vocab

A careaholic is someone who has a strong need to be needed and uses caring and helping in the same way alcoholics use booze to self-medicate pain or cope with stress.

Are You a Careaholic?

Take the quiz in Appendix A called Are You a Careaholic? to see if your caring patterns could be a way to relieve your own stress by using something outside yourself to fix something inside yourself.

My Four-Step Prescription for Stress-Free Helping

William Shakespeare said, "Care is no cure, but rather corrosive for things that are not to be remedied." Don't get me wrong. Helping others is a wonderful thing that makes the world go around. But there's a big difference between stressful caring and compassionate caring. If you take pride in anticipating the needs of others and meeting them before they ask, or if you insist on helping someone—even if they don't want or need your help—you might be taking more than you're giving. You might be feeding your own needs instead of practicing selfless compassion.

You know you're genuinely caring when you have an unselfish desire to give without making others overly dependent on you or taking away their ability to care for themselves. You give only as much help as is really needed. And sometimes you even let people fall down without rescuing them. Here's my prescription to follow for stress-free helping:

➤ Examine your motivations for helping. Do you believe fixing others will fulfill a greater need in you than in them? If the answer is yes, you could be taking more than you're giving. Sometimes the best way to care is not to get involved with someone's problems and not to help them, especially if it robs them of learning and standing on their own two feet.

➤ Respect other people's refusal for your help. It never hurts to let someone know you would like to help. If she says no, it's important to honor the request instead of to pressure her because you see something that needs fixing.

➤ If you end up helping someone, make sure you're in the habit of showing him how to fish instead of feeding him fish. In other words, if the help you give makes someone dependent on you, you're holding him back when he might be ready to be on his own.

➤ Practice what you preach. Before you embark on a helping campaign, help yourself first. Let others benefit from cleaning up their side of the street while you tend to the potholes in your own neglected side. And take time for yourself in the same ways you tell others to care for themselves.

The Doctor Of Calm Is In

We have not really budged a step until we take up residence in someone else's point of view.

—John Erskine

The ability to put yourself in someone's place and see her point of view is easy if she is suffering but much more difficult when her wrath is directed at you. Yet, those who anger you conquer you. My prescription: Think of just one person you can empathize with today, perhaps someone who has done something to upset you. Consider temporarily suspending your point of view (you don't have to give it up for good). Then try to imagine walking around inside that person's body and experiencing the upsetting event in her skin, through her eyes, with her heart—seeing the event from her perspective. I realize this is a bitter pill to swallow, but it's good stress medicine. If you practice this kind of empathy enough, you'll start to notice your stresses dissipating and calmer feelings replacing them. Here's to outsmarting your stress!

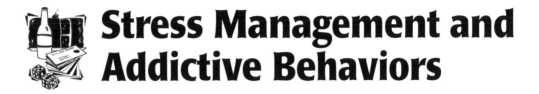

CHAPTER 20

Stress Management and Addictive Behaviors

In This Chapter

➤ What the addictive stress cycle is

➤ Breaking the cycle

➤ Types of addictive behaviors

➤ Hope and help for compulsions and addictions

In this chapter, you'll discover how stress reactions can take the form of addictions and compulsive behaviors in response to unpleasant situations. You'll learn about different types of addictions and how the addictive stress cycle can be broken with exit doors into healthier ways of coping under pressure.

The Addictive Stress Cycle

Stress and addiction go hand in hand. Many people use pick-me-ups to relieve daily pressures—a cup of coffee, a beer, a bowl of ice cream, or a shopping trip. And it's probably safe to say you're no exception. But whether or not your behavior is addictive becomes a matter of degree.

What Are Your Pick-Me-Ups?

Think about what you reach for and how often. Is it booze, pills, or chocolate? Is it occasional or regular? Do you routinely overindulge in alcohol or food? Do you drown yourself in compulsive behaviors such as gambling, spending, sex, or working? Or do you

Stress Vocab

Compulsive behaviors are repetitive and ritualized activities, caused by obsessive thoughts, that help you reduce stress.

know someone who does? Many people relax with a stress reliever on occasion. But if it starts to become a pattern that dominates your life to the exclusion of relationships and responsibilities, listen up. Your compulsive habits can lead to dependency or addiction, serious mental health problems, and broken relationships.

Trending Now from the Smart Files

Here are some statistics on addictions:

➤ The National Institute on Alcohol Abuse and Alcoholism (NIAAA) shows that there are 17.6 million Americans who abuse alcohol or are alcohol dependent.

➤ The National Opinion Research Center reports that an estimated 2.5 million adults are problem gamblers.

➤ Scientists at Stanford University School of Medicine say that chronic overspending is a serious mental health condition for 17 million Americans.

➤ The Society for the Advancement of Sexual Health reports that between 3 and 6 percent of Americans, or 9 million people, have some form of sexual compulsion.

➤ My research team at the University of North Carolina at Charlotte estimates that 25 percent of the American population is workaholic.

When Your Stress "Remedy" Becomes the Problem

Stress nipping at your heels can sink you into an addiction or compulsive habit that locks you into a never-ending prison sentence. If you're already recovering from an addiction and stress pins you against the wall, you're apt to down that drink, lift the spoonful of ice cream, max out your credit cards, overload yourself with work, pick up the needle, or check out the hot flesh online.

Because the "remedy" you use to relieve stress is only temporary, you'll return to it again the next time you're under pressure. When it stops relieving your stress, you'll up the ante, looking for stronger ways to feel good. And you'll need more and more of it each time to feel better. Eventually, the pseudo-remedy that soothed you to begin with becomes the problem. This is called the addictive stress cycle.

Stress Vocab

The addictive stress cycle is the circle that develops when your temporary stress reliever becomes the stressor because your need for it becomes stronger and stronger and you seek more and more of it.

Ten Stages of the Addictive Stress Cycle

Once the addictive pseudo-remedy provides stress relief, although temporary, your natural inclination is to reach for it again and again. Of course, the compulsive habit or addictive behavior doesn't put out the stress firestorm; it only temporarily relieves it, often creating a second-layered problem, addiction. Check out how it breaks down:

➤ Stressor: Stress body slams you or builds up over time.

➤ Self-medication remedy: You reach for the addictive substance or activity to reduce your stressful feelings.

➤ Relief: You temporarily feel calmer along with having a sense of well-being or euphoria.

➤ Self-rebuke: You kick yourself around for giving in to the craving or for falling off the wagon.

➤ Unrealistic promises: You see what happened, promise it won't happen again, and set lofty goals that you'll be perfect next time.

➤ Stressor: Stress builds again, and you miss the good feelings that the addictive pseudo-remedy gave you.

➤ Stinkin' thinkin': Your focus narrows and reaching for the addictive relief seems like the reasonable thing to do, just this one time. And nobody will know but you.

➤ Excuses, excuses: Your mind comes up with a thousand "good reasons" as to why it's okay to use.

➤ You reach for the addictive pseudo-remedy.

➤ Relapse: You're right back where you started.

> ### Truth Serum
>
> Both chemical-based and activity-based addictions follow a similar path:
>
> ➤ Obsessive thoughts
>
> ➤ Uncontrollable compulsive drive
>
> ➤ Going overboard with binges
>
> ➤ Getting the buzz from the dopamine release in the brain during compulsive activity
>
> ➤ Lows from the downward swing, coupled with self-contempt and depression
>
> ➤ Denial and fighting the temptation to reengage in the compulsion, which gradually disintegrates into a relapse, despite disastrous consequences

Here are nine "good reasons" (wink, wink) why it's okay to use:

➤ "I'm tired of depriving myself when I'm hungry."

➤ "I have to work weekends to provide for my family."

➤ "I'm an adult and can have a drink now and then."

➤ "My family doctor prescribed these pills so it's okay."

➤ "I work hard and I deserve to spend a little money on myself."

➤ "A one-night stand now and then won't hurt my marriage."

➤ "I'm just going to watch the poker game for a while."

➤ "Today was a really hard day; I'm gonna take one hit."

➤ "I've thought about it so much I might as well be doing it anyway."

Chemical-Based Addictions

It's helpful to think of addictive behaviors falling into two categories:

➤ Chemical-based addictions such as alcohol, drugs, and food

➤ Activity-based addictions such as compulsive gambling, overspending, compulsive sexual behavior, or workaholism

Addictions, whether chemical or activity based, create a dopamine release in your brain that is associated with compulsive behaviors. You'll remember from Chapter 9 that when released, dopamine creates feelings of euphoria and well-being. Let's start with chemical substances that can lead to addiction when ingested. In this section, we'll cover alcoholism, drug addiction, and food addiction.

The Buzz on Alcoholism and Drug Addiction

How do you know if you're an alcoholic or drug addict? Your alcoholism and drug addiction begins as a way to self-medicate when you're stressed out. You might even tell yourself that you've earned a hit, snort, or drink after your daily grind or spat with your spouse. Eventually, using your drug of choice—alcohol, marijuana, cocaine, or other substance— starts to snowball into dependence, then into an inability to stop.

You insist that your boss, spouse, or coworkers are the reasons for your substance abuse. You downplay its negative aspects, accuse friends and loved ones of exaggerating, and refuse to take responsibility for your actions. You tell them you wouldn't use if they'd get off your back and that you can quit anytime. But your compulsion to use overtakes your rational understanding of the damage you've done neglecting your health, relationships, personal finances, and career.

You might graduate to cocaine or methamphetamines, which trigger a dopamine release in your brain. Over time, you develop a tolerance and need for a greater amount of drugs and alcohol to get the same effects. During the chemically induced high, you feel like the world's biggest "bad ass." You have blackouts that make you forget who you were with or what you were doing while you were stoned. As the euphoria wears off, you go through withdrawal from the substance. Your mind is foggy, and you have a headache and experience nausea, sweating, shakiness, anxiety, and loss of appetite.

The Buzz on Food Addiction

How do you know if you're a food addict? You have an urge to eat compulsively. When you're down in the dumps, you notice that sweets and salty junk foods comfort and numb you. You have become physiologically and mentally dependent upon sugar, flour, and wheat substances. You have a biochemical disease. Thoughts of food, excessive cravings, and obsessions to eat dominate your mind. And the uncontrollable act of locating and consuming food trumps other aspects of your life.

You gorge yourself in private, hoard a large amount of food, and hide your eating binges from others. When you binge, eating from containers and drinking out of cartons, you lose count of how much you've consumed. As you continue to stuff yourself, you fall into an eating trance that numbs you from stress and worry. But you deny that you have a biochemical disease and believe if you tried harder or developed more willpower you could lick the bad eating habits. You promise you'll clean up your act by counting calories, yo-yo dieting, eliminating carbs, or joining Weight Watchers. But you get so weary of denying yourself food pleasures that you give up trying altogether. You turn to comfort foods and trigger foods—chocolate, potato chips, or fill in the blank—become your consoler.

Truth Serum

Eating highs come from binges on salt, sugar, and starches (sugar incognito)—substances that are immediately metabolized and turned into sugar in your bloodstream. In addition to the dopamine release in your brain, studies show that certain proteins in foods such as wheat or milk contain narcotic-like painkillers.

During a food rush, you notice that your senses are heightened and your emotions are more intense and irrational. Even if you suffer from dangerous health conditions such as diabetes or heart disease and you know the deadly consequences, your cravings for sugar and carbs (the trigger foods that make you ill) win the battle. Your intimate relationships, social interactions, and career take a back seat to obtaining and consuming addictive foods.

Activity-Based Addictions

It's harder for you to detect addiction when it looks like an ordinary activity such as shopping or working that you engage in regularly. Getting activity addictions recognized as serious problems has been an uphill battle.

You might brag about being a workaholic and wear the badge proudly. Or you might chuckle about being a shopaholic, tossing around the phrase, "shop 'til you drop." These compulsive behaviors are real problems that can destroy your personal life and relationships and even lead to health problems and financial ruin.

The Buzz on Compulsive Gambling

How do you know if you're a compulsive gambler? Your thoughts of gambling create a stimulation and excitement that help you escape from escalating stress and worry. Gambling and thoughts of gambling dominate your life to the exclusion of everything else. Acting on your uncontrollable urge to gamble reduces your restlessness and irritability and puts you in a trancelike state that numbs your impulse control.

Truth Serum

Studies show that it's the risk of winning or losing that heightens pleasure centers in the brain and drives the preoccupation with gaming and the anticipation of winning. Over time, you raise the stakes to maintain your rush. The heightened excitement from high-risk bets at the casino, lottery, racetrack, or with a bookie put you in a position of losing everything. And eventually you do lose—big time.

Losses are followed by a downward swing of remorse and blaming others. Compulsive gambling is linked to a high rate of financial ruin, domestic violence, and divorce. Of the cash wagered in casinos, 40 to 60 percent is withdrawn at ATMs from personal accounts or as cash advances from credit cards.

Over time, you increase the frequency of wagers, despite mounting personal debt, career jeopardy, and family unrest. One win and you feel an extreme sense of power and control. Your feelings of omnipotence tell you that more betting will yield even greater rewards. So you continue gambling around the clock. Despite financial ruin, you convince yourself that your luck will change. Even though your losses outweigh your wins, you remember your winnings more than your losses. You chase your losses, convinced you'll win them back. But your continued betting descends you further into debt and family deterioration.

The Buzz on Compulsive Spending

How do you know if you have a spending addiction? Fantasies of shopping and spending dominate your thinking and block your stress and worry. You act on your uncontrollable urge to spend so that you can reduce your stress. You go on spending sprees making purchases that you can't afford, don't need, and will never use. The spending trance eclipses the reality of

Truth Serum

Retail excursions jolt a dose of dopamine (the same chemical your body releases during sex and cocaine use) to your brain and give you a short-lived high. Spending gives you feelings of power and control that momentarily bring you out of the worry-stress doldrums. After you tally your credit card bills and realize your life is in shambles, you feel deep remorse, shame, and depression.

Compulsive spenders suffer from abnormally high levels of depression, anxiety, and mood disorders, and their relationships and careers are put in jeopardy.

your spending problem: you're already drowning in debt, and your closets and drawers are bulging with merchandise, price tags still attached, from previous retail splurges.

You can't control the compulsion to spend. You minimize your problem, criticize loved ones for magnifying it, and refuse to admit you're out of control. The only way to comfort your self-contempt and resentment is to recapture that good feeling when you spend. Soon you'll be right back on the Internet, the shopping channel, or in the mall spending money you don't have, buying items you don't need, and hiding purchases from your bewildered family.

The Buzz on Compulsive Sexual Behavior

How do you know if you have a sexual addiction? Sexual thoughts dominate your mind and you fantasize of varied and frequent sexual acts, usually as a release from obsessive worry or job pressures.

Truth Serum

Your rush comes from the anticipation of sexual conquests and high-risk sexual activity. You feel no true intimate connection with your sexual partners, and maintaining anonymity heightens the excitement. The sex act itself jolts you with the same dopamine dose that cocaine gives. In some cases your need for greater risk leads you into illegal activities such as exhibitionism, obscene phone calls, voyeurism, or sex in public places. Eventually, an arrest, a health crisis, a crumbling marriage, or job loss causes you to hit bottom. You feel self-contempt for the extremes your sexual behaviors have taken and the shambles your life is in.

You organize your world around sexual activity to the exclusion of all other aspects of life, looking for sex wherever you can find it. You get temporary relief from sexually acting out in ways that often have negative or dangerous consequences: unsafe anonymous sex, surfing the web for one-night stands, cybersex, Internet pornography, multiple sexual partners, extramarital affairs, strip clubs, phone sex, massage parlors, and compulsive masturbation. Studies show that more than 25 percent of those with Internet access view pornography during work hours.

The Buzz on Workaholism

How do you know if you're a workaholic? You're on the ski slopes dreaming about working on your computer. You can't stop thinking about, talking about, or engaging in work. Your work projects take priority over every other aspect of your life. Your uncontrollable urge to work engulfs you in a work fog that numbs you to your anxiety, worry, and stress, and to other people.

Truth Serum

You don't need drugs because your bloodstream is manufacturing its own crystal meth. You're an adrenaline junkie, moaning about things moving too slowly and the shortage of time. You put yourself under pressure, unable to catch up with work demands. Your buzz comes from adrenaline-charged binge working after you set unrealistic deadlines that throw you into a cycle of toiling around the clock, hurrying and rushing, and multitasking to get to the finish line. Work euphoria eventually gives way to work hangovers: withdrawal, depression, irritability, and anxiety.

Studies that I conducted at the University of North Carolina at Charlotte show across the board that workaholics, compared to non-workaholics, have higher stress levels and burnout rates, less self-insight, greater communication problems, and more controlling personalities.

You get soused by overloading yourself with more tasks than you can possibly complete. You work nonstop for days on end—morning to night, weekends, and holidays—instead of spreading out work projects over time. You throw all-nighters to meet self-imposed deadlines, sometimes sleeping off a work binge in your clothes.

Preoccupation with work puts you into a work trance or brownouts that take you out of the present moment, causing you to forget conversations, misplace things, or lose your train of thought. Your 24/7 electronic devices keep you connected to work and disconnected from people.

Risky Business: How to Spot a Workaholic

Rate your boss, spouse, best friend, or yourself using the test in Appendix A called Risky Business: How to Spot a Workaholic.

Breaking the Addictive Cycle

Nowadays many resources are available to help you break a compulsive habit or addiction. But there's no one-size-fits-all solution. In more serious cases, you might need a support group or professional help to achieve successful recovery. But you might be able to kick a bad habit like overspending, overeating, or overworking on your own.

Have a Relapse-Prevention Plan

Whether you're struggling with gambling, overspending, or alcoholism, or you're simply trying to quit smoking, having a relapse-prevention plan makes the difference between succeeding or throwing in the towel. A relapse-prevention plan is a self-made solution that states "if a risky or tempting situation occurs, then I'll respond in a predetermined way."

You'll remember from earlier chapters that the built-in strategy of the if-then plan inoculates you from the impulsive what-the-hell attitude: "If I'm in a bad mood, I'll call my sponsor or go to an AA meeting," or "If I feel like I want a cigarette, I'll chew a piece of Nicorette," or "If I overshoot my budget, I'll be compassionate with myself and stop spending immediately."

Shock Absorber

Setbacks are a natural part of moving forward. Just know ahead of time that a relapse is possible. Above all, refrain from self-rebuke if you have a setback. And make sure you use self-compassion to offset any compulsive need to comfort your disappointment by returning to your drug of choice. If you fall off the wagon, pick yourself up, brush yourself off, and take another step forward.

Making a U-Turn

You can intervene on yourself at any point in the addiction cycle through exit doors that break the spiraling. First, you pay attention to where you are in the cycle. Once you identify the stage you're in, you can engage in a healthy activity to reduce your stress. This could be attending a 12-Step meeting such as Alcoholics Anonymous or Spenders Anonymous (see Appendix B for contact information for 12-Step programs), calling a support person, reading a daily inspirational passage, or some other activity in your preset recovery plan.

Facing Compulsive Infidelity

Once you start bootlegging your compulsion, you might as well face it: you're desperate. You feel you must practice your addiction at all costs, even if it means being deceitful and dishonest, even if it hurts the ones you love the most. Here are some examples:

➤ The compulsive gambler on the sly withdraws thousands of dollars from a joint checking account to bet at the racetrack.

➤ The compulsive spender stashes bulging shopping bags in a secret location that her husband doesn't know about.

➤ The sex addict masturbates to live sex on the Internet while his wife sleeps in the next room.

➤ The workaholic sneaks work projects on vacation because he's wedded to work.

Now that you realize your problem is out of control and it's time to take action, here are some steps to keep any compulsive infidelity from swindling you out of a happy, productive life:

➤ Stay on top of your compulsive behavior and keep accounts of it. Most people say they weren't aware of how often they engaged in overeating, overspending, overworking (you fill in the blank). But when you keep a record of how much and how often, the extent of the compulsion becomes clear. And your own records can be sobering enough to wake you up.

➤ Develop a policy to reign in your actions. Abstaining from alcohol or drug abuse is clear, but abstaining from activity addictions such as overworking or overspending is more nebulous. It requires a work plan or spending plan that has built-in limits on the behavior.

➤ Substitute healthier outlets for your compulsion and engage in activities that allow you to vent your stress and release tension.

➤ Confide your compulsive infidelity to a trusted friend, loved one, clergy, support group, or professional instead of carrying the burden of shame and guilt, which only fuels the addiction.

➤ Practice some of the stress-reduction strategies such as deep breathing and meditation discussed in earlier chapters to neutralize the addictive cycle.

➤ Take care of yourself physically and emotionally by making sure you get the basics: ample rest, exercise, and nutrition. Put balance back in your life with family time, play, work, social relationships, spirituality, and time for yourself.

➤ Block out refueling time to clear your mind and get to know yourself on the inside through inspirational readings, prayer, meditation, or contemplation. See if you can get to the underlying causes of your compulsive behavior.

➤ Trump your immediate gratification by setting long-term goals of where you want to go in life. Stick to your road map. If you continue to detour, get outside help.

➤ Consider professional help if you find it impossible to follow through with any of these suggestions. Sometimes compulsive infidelity is too difficult to manage alone, and medication and counseling are needed.

12-Step Programs and Recovery

Breaking the addiction cycle cannot always be done alone.

Addiction is the result of external relief winning out over your inner resources to manage stress. In recovery, you focus on your inner life—feelings, understandings, insights, and simply getting to know yourself better. Once you have more clarity, serenity, strength, and stability within yourself, your life starts to unfold in a parallel manner and direction. When you're calm and stable from the inside out, calmness and stability will embrace you from the outside in.

The Twelve Steps

The Twelve Steps have worked for millions of people with a variety of addictions, including alcohol and other drugs, food, gambling, shopping, work, sex, and addictive relationships. These Steps are vehicles for healing bad habits, compulsions, and addictions and establishing a more meaningful and fulfilling life:

> ➤ We admitted we were powerless over (name your compulsion)—that our lives had become unmanageable.

> ➤ We came to believe that a power greater than ourselves could restore us to sanity.

> ➤ We made a decision to turn our will and our lives over to the care of God as we understood God.

> ➤ We made a searching and fearless moral inventory of ourselves.

> ➤ We admitted to God, to ourselves, and to another human being the exact nature of our wrongs.

> ➤ We were entirely ready to have God remove all these defects of character.

> ➤ We humbly asked God to remove our shortcomings.

> ➤ We made a list of all persons we had harmed and became willing to make amends to them all.

> ➤ We made direct amends to such people whenever possible, except when to do so would injure them or others.

> ➤ We continued to take personal inventory and when we were wrong, we promptly admitted it.

➤ We sought through prayer and meditation to improve our conscious contact with God *as we understood God*, praying only for knowledge of God's will for us and the power to carry that out.

➤ Having had a spiritual awakening as the result of these Steps, we tried to carry this message to others, and to practice these principles in all our affairs.

Spiritual Practices

The Twelve Steps are not religious. They are spiritual practices that refer to the God or higher power of your own understanding instead of a specific religious prescription. These practices involve letting go of absolute control by "accepting the things you cannot change, changing the things you can, and having the wisdom to know the difference." They include accepting your strengths and limitations, being willing to change through patience one step at a time, tolerating uncertainty, and focusing on your progress instead of on perfection.

12-Step Programs

Although the Twelve Steps originated with Alcoholics Anonymous, you can apply them to recovery from any compulsion or addiction. If you find that you're not able to break your compulsive behavior, it might require outside help. You can find a 12-Step support group in your area by going online. These groups meet often, are free and available in major US cities. Appendix B contains names of the major 12-Step programs and their website addresses.

The Doctor Of Calm Is In

God grant me the serenity to accept the things I cannot change, the courage to change the things I can, and the wisdom to know the difference

—Reinhold Niebuhr

This simple but profound prayer has helped millions of people deal with their compulsions. In times of strain, citing this prayer to yourself can bring you great calm and serenity. My prescription: This age-old prayer is good medicine for your parasympathetic nervous system. When you're upset over things you cannot control, say the "Serenity Prayer" quietly to yourself until you feel calm and stress symptoms fall away. Here's to outsmarting your stress!

CHAPTER 21

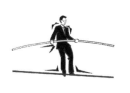

Maintaining Work-Life Balance and Stress Resilience

In This Chapter

➤ Evaluating your work-life balance

➤ Finding your resilient zone

➤ Tips for maintaining stress resilience

In this chapter, you'll get a chance to evaluate your work-life balance and then develop a stress-proof plan based on your findings. You'll also discover your resilient zone, along with fifty ways to leave stress behind and maintain stress resilience in your life.

Work-Life Balance

Music artists have long known something about work-life balance that most of the world still doesn't get. Cyndi Lauper sang it: "When the workin' day is done / Oh girls they wanna have fun." Michael Jackson crooned it in *Off the Wall*: "So tonight / Gotta leave that nine to five upon the shelf / An' just enjoy yourself." What about you? Are you able to leave personal problems and job worries behind, have fun, and fully engage in your life?

Trending Now from the Smart Files

Here are some statistics on work-life balance:

➤ A team of Canadian and American researchers found that nearly half of US workers take work home with them and many of them say it interferes with family, social, and leisure aspects of their lives. Workers toiling more than fifty hours a week have the most interference in their personal lives.

➤ According to a *New York Times*/CBS News poll, 40 percent of people under forty-five say they check work e-mails after hours or on vacations; one in seven say electronic devices cut time spent with spouses, and one in ten say these devices cut time spent with their children.

➤ Studies show that 30 percent of Americans say they have trouble coping with work stress while vacationing, and 19 percent postpone or cancel vacations for work-related reasons.

Shrinkage of Personal Time

Today, more than ever, the average American is challenged with finding a work-life balance. According to a CareerBuilder poll, 44 percent of working moms say work preoccupies them at home. And 37 percent of working dads bring work home at least one day a week; 30 percent work most weekends.

With more things to do and life moving faster, you, too, might feel that your personal time is shrinking. If you add to that a technologically driven culture that has erased the line that once protected private hours, your work-life balance is at risk.

Chances are you're stretching long hours to juggle more tasks, taking work home, leashing yourself to wireless electronics, making yourself available 24/7, and giving up much-needed vacation time. Living this way keeps your natural defenses on high alert, marinating you in your stress juices (cortisol and adrenaline), and clobbering you with mental and physical illnesses.

Keep Your Stress Tools on Speed Dial

Everybody has a breaking point with this kind of stress. The goal is to realize you've hit yours long before symptoms set in. So listen to your body when it's tired or burned out, and take time out to respond to the stress signals. That's when it's time to slip in some of the stress cushions you've mastered in the course of the book: deep breathing, relaxation techniques, mindful awareness, meditation, visualizations, the pendulum, positive self-talk, or reframing to name a few. And you can practice them lying in bed before you get up, in the shower, commuting to work, on your lunch break, standing in line, waiting at the doctor's office, stuck in traffic, and before drifting off to sleep. There's always a time and place to cushion the pressures of the day.

Recharging Your Batteries

Denying yourself the segue from a stressful workday to free time keeps your stress alarm on overtime and puts stress overload on your body. Consider using your commute time from office to home to decompress from the day's pressures instead of chewing over stressful events. Play enjoyable music, engage in relaxation exercises, practice mindful open awareness of the views around you, yawn and stretch, or just let your mind linger in the sweetness of doing nothing. These cushions will refuel you to enter the next phase of your day with renewed energy.

Is Your Busy Signal Green, Yellow, or Red?

Some people get so addicted to their adrenaline rush that they gravitate to high-pressure jobs and keep piling on new work tasks. Do you stress yourself with overwork, or are you just a plain hard worker? Rate yourself on your work habits with the test in Appendix A called Risky Business: How to Spot a Workaholic.

Truth Serum

Studies show that major businesses hire workaholics because they think they'll get a bigger bang for their buck. But research shows workaholics don't make the best workers. The rate of burnout is higher, the trajectory of their careers is lower, and they are not team players.

My own research at the University of North Carolina at Charlotte shows greater marital estrangement in marriages of workaholics. And workaholics are 40 percent more likely to end up divorced. Plus, children of workaholics have a higher rate of anxiety and depression than children of non-workaholics.

What's Out of Whack?

Regardless of how you scored on the Risky Business test, chances are your goal is the same as most people's: to achieve and maintain a balanced, stress-free life. But how do you get there? Achieving balance is sometimes a tightwire act, but the work-life inventory can help. One way to view your life is to think of it as a wheel made up of four spokes.

The Four Spokes of Life

➤ Work: Healthy work habits include being effective and productive on the job, enjoying what you do for a living, working harmoniously with coworkers, and working moderately while giving equal time to other areas of your life.

➤ Family: Your family includes positive communication and communion with your partner and other loved ones. In today's world, family configuration means many different things to different people. Your family can be you and your spouse and can include your children. It can include single parents with children, unmarried partners who cohabitate, gay and lesbian couples with or without children, or adults who reside with older parents or siblings.

➤ Play: The play spoke extends your need for social interaction outside your family to friendships and social pastimes. Play consists of fun activities you participate in for pure enjoyment—recreational activities or volunteer work that takes you away from your everyday routines and stressors.

➤ Self: Last but not least is the self, often considered last and least important. The self spoke includes personal needs you meet by taking good care of yourself. A few examples are spiritual nurturance, meditation, relaxation, nutrition, sleep, exercise, and various and sundry guilty pleasures and indulgences.

Each spoke is valued equally and gets equal attention if your wheel is balanced enough to hold its shape. If one quadrant is unattended, the circle starts to deflate, loses its shape, and becomes lopsided. Few people are perfectly balanced. But the closer you come to fullness, the less stressed and more alive you feel as a human being.

The Work-Life Inventory

The work-life inventory can help you discover if balance is missing in one or more of your life spokes. Then you can use this knowledge to develop your own personal stress-proof plan.

Using the rating scale of 1: never true, 2: seldom true, 3: often true, and 4: always true, put the number that best fits you in the blank beside each statement. For your total score, add the eight numbers and put the sum in the blank at the end of the area.

Spoke 1: Work

___I have many interests outside work.

___I spend as much time after hours with family and friends as I do with coworkers.

___I enjoy my work today as much as ever, and I am productive and effective at what I do.

___I work overtime only on special occasions.

___I'm able to leave my work at the workplace.

___I'm good at organizing and pacing my work time so that it doesn't interfere with other commitments.

___I work moderately, pace myself, and confine my job to regular working hours.

___I spend an equal amount of time relaxing and socializing with friends as I do working.

___Total Work Score

Spoke 2: Family

___I communicate well with members of my family.

___I take an active interest in the lives of other family members.

___My family spends quality time together.

___My family plays together and takes outings regularly.

___I participate actively in family celebrations, traditions, and rituals.

___I have good interpersonal relationships with other family members.

___I enjoy spending time with my family.

___My family and work lives are in harmony with each other.

___Total Family Score

Spoke 3: Play

___I socialize with friends who are not coworkers.

___I enjoy social gatherings.

___I participate in recreational activities that help me unwind and relax.

___I go out socially with friends.

___My social life and work life are in harmony with each other.

___I enjoy inviting friends to my house for dinner.

___I like social pastimes where I can relax with friends.

___It feels good to laugh, have fun, and get my mind off work.

___Total Play Score

Spoke 4: Self

___I plan time each day just for me to do whatever I want.

___For fun I have a hobby or pastime I enjoy.

___I regularly take time out for meditation, prayer, contemplation, inspirational reading, church or synagogue attendance, 12-Step meetings, or other spiritual activity.

___I eat nutritional, well-balanced meals.

___I make sure I get adequate rest and sleep.

___I make time for weekly physical exercise.

___I am optimistic and try to see the best in myself.

___I make sure I get my personal needs met.

___**Total Self Score**

Your Balance Wheel of Life

On the balance wheel that follows, put an X on the number of each spoke that corresponds with your total score. Draw a line from that number to the center of the wheel. Then darken the entire area of the circle from your total score back to the number 8.

For example, if your total self score is 16, put an X over the number 16 in the self spoke of the wheel. Draw a line from 16 to the center of the circle; darken that area from the center outward between 8 and 16. Repeat these steps for all four spokes of the wheel. The part of the wheel with the biggest shaded spoke is the one in which you are most balanced. The spoke that is less complete is the area of your life that needs attention.

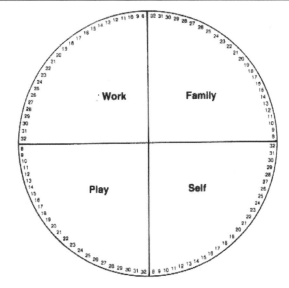

Figure: Your Balance Wheel of Life

Keeping an Even Keel

When you look at your balance wheel, you'll see that there are things you can do to establish and maintain balance and keep stress at bay. What do you notice? What do you like or dislike about what you see? And what do you want to change? How would you do it and when will you begin?

Shock Absorber

One way to create clear boundaries between work and your personal life is to carry a separate cell phone for the job. Use a laptop for work and a desktop for home to keep the lines clearly drawn. If you have an in-home office, treat it as if it's five miles away. Go there only when you work, and keep the door closed after hours. Another way to draw the line between work and off-time is to ask yourself if you had a "to be" list alongside your "to do" list what would it look like? (one example might be sitting outdoors, listening to nature sounds). Jot down your "to be" list in your stress journal.

Developing a Stress-Proof Plan

After reviewing your wheel and thinking about the questions, set some goals for each spoke that will help you achieve more balance and reduce your stress level. Putting your goals into practice becomes the basis for your stress-proof plan. After you try your plan for a while, periodically revise it with what you want to keep, add, or delete. In the spaces below, list your goals for each spoke after the examples I've provided to get you started:

Work example: I will set boundaries around the number of hours I work this week by taking my lunch break and avoiding work e-mails and phone calls after 6:00 pm.

Family example: I will plan extra time to have fun with my loved ones.

Play example: I will develop one new social pastime totally unrelated to work.

Self example: I will practice stress-relief exercises by meditating for fifteen minutes each morning and working out three times a week.

Recharging Your Batteries

Here are some reminders to help you hit the bull's-eye with your plan: Arrange to power down and clock out at a certain time. Don't take work home with you unless it's the exception and only when absolutely necessary. Learn to say no and draw the line when someone asks you to do something you don't have time for. If you have to add a new task, knock another one off your to-do list so you don't get overloaded. Tell yourself there is a limit to what you can do and put the rest out of the picture.

Whatever Happened to Spare Time?

A 2008 Gallup Poll found that 54 percent of Americans say they don't have enough spare time and that this state of affairs frequently causes them stress. Where does the time go? Why isn't there enough time left over just for you, time for fun and relaxation? This exercise can help you understand how you use your time and think about how you can rearrange your life in order to include time for yourself. Fill in the number of hours you spend each day in the following activities:

Hours Per Day Activity

M   T   W   Th   F   Sa   Su

___ ___ ___ ___ ___ ___ ___ Sleeping

___ ___ ___ ___ ___ ___ ___ Eating

___ ___ ___ ___ ___ ___ ___ Household chores such as cleaning, cooking, washing dishes

___ ___ ___ ___ ___ ___ ___ Running errands

___ ___ ___ ___ ___ ___ ___ Preparing for work

___ ___ ___ ___ ___ ___ ___ Studying

___ ___ ___ ___ ___ ___ ___ Getting to and from work

___ ___ ___ ___ ___ ___ ___ Working

___ ___ ___ ___ ___ ___ ___ Taking care of other family members

___ ___ ___ ___ ___ ___ ___ Social or family obligations

___ ___ ___ ___ ___ ___ ___ Volunteer or civic work

___ ___ ___ ___ ___ ___ ___ Carpooling or chauffeuring

168 hours

___ Total Activity Hours per Week

___ Spare Time

There are 168 hours in a week. Subtract your total activity hours from this number to get the number of hours left over for spare time to do the things you really want to do. Then answer the following questions in your stress journal:

➤ What has this exercise told me about how I'm living my life?

➤ What can I glean about how I spend my time through the week?

➤ How can I change my life for more *being* and less *doing?*

➤ How can I distribute my remaining hours over the week to give myself more spare time?

Stress Vocab

Stress resilience is your ability to face challenges, accept them, and keep on going through the stressors.

Maintaining Stress Resilience

Hopefully, by now you have a greater understanding of how to use time and balance to create a more stress-free life. Armed with this information, you can maintain stress resilience over the long haul. Let's look at some ways to accomplish this.

Finding Your Resilient Zone

How do you get to your resilient zone and then maintain it? Your ability to create a resilient zone hangs on several factors. Take a look:

➤ The strain of having others dependent upon you

➤ The number and frequency of traumatic events you've faced

➤ Outside pressures

➤ The degree of your responsibilities and commitments

➤ Strong supportive relationships

➤ Your ability to take care of yourself

➤ Your overall physical health

➤ A positive outlook

You can control some of these factors while others are beyond your control. But when you focus on the resources you have at your fingertips, instead of the limitations, you've found your resilient zone: staying healthy, getting ample sleep, exercising, eating well, drawing on your optimism, establishing strong social contacts, and limiting outside pressures. It doesn't matter how much money or education you have. To find your resilient zone, you dwell on your resources instead of your losses. You reach out to others, stay in touch with loved ones, and volunteer to help when and where you can.

On the flip side, the route to your resilient zone is through stepping into the unfamiliar and unexpected. I realize this sounds contradictory, but it's one of life's paradoxes: you build stress resilience by having a degree of control while embracing novelty. You're more likely to find your resilient zone if you stick your neck out than if you settle into ruts and routines. Try new things—such as meet different people, develop a new skill, learn a new game, or travel to a new place. So ask yourself what you can add or change—no matter how small—to spice up your life.

Fifty Ways to Maintain Stress Resilience

There are probably as many old wives' tales about how to relieve stress as there are for removing warts. Inspired by Paul Simon's "Fifty Ways to Leave Your Lover," I've come up with fifty ways to leave stress behind and maintain resilience. Mine are backed up by science, serving as summary reminders of the main points in the book.

> ➤ Manage your electronic devices instead of letting them manage you.

> ➤ Celebrate important milestones (such as birthdays and anniversaries) in your life.

> ➤ Stay in the here and now as much as you can.

> ➤ Take your vacations or at the very least staycations.

> ➤ Leave space in your schedule for heart-to-heart talks with people you care about.

> ➤ Insert stress cushions wherever you can so that stress doesn't metastasize into your life.

> ➤ Unwind from a stressful day by listening to soothing music.

> ➤ Practice progressive muscle relaxation, the relaxation response, and deep breathing to stay stress resistant.

> ➤ Make meditation, yoga, prayer, or contemplation an integral part of your daily regimen.

> ➤ Carry realistic expectations of yourself and others.

> ➤ Balance hard work with play, family time, and self-care.

> ➤ Keep a "to be" list alongside your "to do" list.

> ➤ Give yourself pep talks and be kind, calm, and supportive.

> ➤ Be mindful of eating, talking, and walking slowly.

> ➤ Maintain an optimistic attitude and focus on solutions instead of problems.

> ➤ Stick your neck out and face challenges that broaden you.

> ➤ Avoid stressful situations that impede your growth.

> ➤ Nurture yourself with good nutrition, vigorous exercise, and ample sleep (at least six hours or more a night).

> ➤ Look for common ground in all your relationships.

> ➤ Enjoy sex with your intimate partner as often as you both want.

> ➤ Spend as much time as you can in nature and bring as much inside as possible.

➤ Volunteer or do something for someone else to take your mind off your worries and improve your stress health.

➤ Pay close attention to the attitude you bring to the office each day and keep it in check from time to time.

➤ Ask yourself how you're treating stress instead of how stress is treating you.

➤ Show self-compassion—not self-pity—when the going gets rough.

Shock Absorber

When you take a bird's eye view of your life, it gives you an objective perspective, an outsider's slant on ways to maintain stress resilience and a healthy balance. If getting away from your everyday environment isn't possible, spend one day going through your routines, imagining that you're viewing them through the eyes of an outsider. As you move through your day, note what you see with curiosity, as if it's a first-time experience. Is it the stress of another pressure cooker day or exciting challenges that lie ahead? Do you crack the whip or treat yourself with kindness? Are you enslaved by cell phones, iPads, or laptops, or do you master your electronics by taking time to see what's going on around you with renewed interest? Do you sneer at other people who don't move fast enough, or are you more tolerant of their unique style?

After going through this exercise, notice if you have a renewed appreciation for life. Then write about your impressions in your stress journal.

➤ Be on the lookout for mind traps that you can fall into and actions you can take to get out of them.

➤ Think of stress as a friend trying to protect you instead of an enemy working against you.

➤ Avoid using alcohol, drugs, food, or work to relieve stress.

➤ Take up hobbies and fun pastimes that take your mind off your daily pressures.

➤ Pamper yourself from time to time with a massage, manicure, facial, pedicure, or some other guilty pleasure.

➤ Stress-proof your home and make it a sanctuary from daily pressures.

➤ Enjoy the companionship of a pet to calm you down.

➤ Know the difference between imagined and real threats.

➤ Distinguish between the stressors you can and can't change, change the ones you can, and accept those beyond your control.

➤ Repeat the gratitude exercise often.

➤ Maintain a strong support group of friends, family, neighbors, and coworkers.

➤ Ask yourself if there's anything about your perspective you can change to lighten your stress load.

➤ Unplug by taking power naps during the day.

➤ Roll with the punches instead of having a "stressfest" over the little curveballs life throws at you.

➤ Try to find something in stressful events that you can learn and grow from.

➤ Make commitments to things bigger than yourself such as team spirit and the common good.

➤ Familiarize yourself with your stress coping style and modify anything that works against your stress resilience.

➤ Know what your inner resources are and when to ratchet them up.

➤ Stack your positivity deck by looking at the flip side of a negative situation.

➤ Take short breaks in the course of your day.

➤ Tickle your funny bone often with jokes, light-hearted humor, and laughter.

➤ Practice the art of empathy to neutralize anger and frustration and bring you stress relief.

➤ Don't let your mind's negativity bias cause you to overestimate threats and underestimate your resources.

➤ Get in the habit of taking your stress temperature and lowering it with some of the stress relievers from the book.

➤ Choose your battles; tell yourself, "I can overcome anything I set my mind to." And above all, never give up.

"Push-Throughs" for Building Resilience

No matter how great the stress, there's always a "push through" to keep you stress resistant. Push-throughs empower you with the feeling of pressing outward against stress instead of feeling stress pressing inward upon you.

You can tackle some stressors head-on. If a coworker snaps at you, say you don't like to be spoken to that way. Find ways around stress instead of crumbling under it. If the game is rained out, you can throw a party instead of a fit. There are times when it pays to sidestep stressful situations. If loud music freaks you out, avoid Lady Gaga concerts.

When all else fails, change your outlook. If you're hit with a big tax debt, remind yourself that you made more money than ever.

The Doctor Of Calm Is In

Our greatest weapon against stress is our ability to choose one thought over another

—William James

You have more power over stress than you think. A lot of resilience comes from the attitude you take toward your stressors and the knowledge that you always have choices. My prescription: Next time stress slugs you, face it head-on, go around it, dodge it, or change your outlook. And you won't have to take an aspirin and call me in the morning. Here's to outsmarting your stress and maintaining resilience over the long haul!

When You're Cortisol Drenched: A Final Word

Life is full of possibilities that allow you to maintain stress resilience long after reading this book. When you take your stress temperature from time to time and discover you're cortisol drenched, activate the stress-resilient strategies you've mastered so far. Better yet, employ one final tool to prevent stress from sneaking up on you: my favorite poem by Portia Nelson, "An Autobiography in Five Short Chapters."

On any given day, read this poem to see the water you're swimming in before you get snared in the stress of your life. Then peek inside yourself with a curious eye, and ask which chapter you're in and if you need to take another course of action by walking down another street.

An Autobiography in Five Short Chapters

Chapter I
I walk down the street.
There is a deep hole in the sidewalk.
I fall in.

I am lost . . . I am helpless.
It isn't my fault.
It takes forever to find a way out.

Chapter II
I walk down the same street.
There is a deep hole in the sidewalk.
I pretend I don't see it.
I fall in again.
I can't believe I am in the same place.
But, it isn't my fault.
It still takes a long time to get out.

Chapter III
I walk down the same street.
There is a deep hole in the sidewalk.
I see it is there.
I still fall in . . . it's a habit.
My eyes are open.
I know where I am.
It is my fault.
I get out immediately.

Chapter IV
I walk down the same street.
There is a deep hole in the sidewalk.
I walk around it.

Chapter V
I walk down another street.

Endings

It can be difficult to see that just as the Phoenix rises from the ashes, we are always ending and beginning, all at the same time: saying good-bye, completing a class, ending a job or relationship. With endings, the loss can overshadow the gains, but they have their bright side too. On New Year's Eve you can feel nostalgic about the past year and make enthusiastic resolutions for the new one. The end of summer shepherds in the beginning of fall. The ending of this book brings an opportunity for you to practice the stress techniques contained here and a chance to reread portions that were meaningful.

The poet T.S. Eliot said it best when he wrote, "What we call the beginning is often the end. And to make an end is to make a beginning. The end is where we start from."

PART SIX

Resources for Further Managing Stress

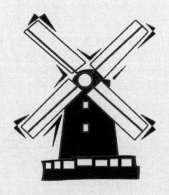

APPENDIX A

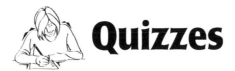 **Quizzes**

In This Appendix

➤ Quizzes

➤ Score Guides

In this appendix, you'll find quizzes that will help you evaluate yourself on various stress-related issues, from looking at the way you use electronic devices to assessing the stress level of your workplace. Your self-evaluations give you a thumbnail sketch of where you stand on stress issues compared to other people. Based on your scores, related chapters provide tips on what actions you can take to outsmart stress and develop stress-resilience.

Do Your Wireless Leashes Have a Choke Hold on You? (from Chapter 3)

To compute your choke hold score, answer yes or no to the following questions:

____1. Do you have one or more wireless devices with you most of the time?

____2. When you're away from your workplace, is it hard for you to stop using them?

____3. Do you feel antsy in situations where you cannot use a wireless device?

____4. Have you ever slept with (or close to) one or more wireless devices so you won't miss out on something?

____5. Do you usually interrupt conversations with loved ones and/or friends to respond to electronic gadgets?

___6. Do you usually continue texting or e-mailing after your coworkers, friends, or family members have called it quits?

___7. Is checking your devices one of the last things you do before bedtime?

___8. Is checking your devices one of the first things you do when you wake up in the morning?

___9. Have your wireless devices ever created problems in your personal relationships?

___10. Do you prefer to spend more time with your wireless devices than socializing or hanging out with friends and family?

___11. Would it be easy for you to remove electronic devices from your life?

___12. Is it easy for you to ignore them after the workday ends?

___13. Are you able to relax and enjoy life in the slow lane without your cell phone or laptop?

___14. Is it easy for you to leave your devices behind when you go on vacation?

___15. Would it be a snap for you to go a whole workday without using one?

___16. Most of the time do you put your devices out of sight, out of mind after work hours?

___17. Generally, do you silence them during a workday when you're interacting with people?

___18. Does it bother you in public places when other people check their devices in close earshot of you?

___19. Do you believe multitasking with wireless devices can create problems in your life?

___20. Do you prefer face-to-face interactions with colleagues and clients over electronic communication?

How to Calculate Your Score

To calculate your choke hold score, start with 60 points. Subtract 2 points for each yes answer and add 2 points for each no answer to questions 1–10. Subtract 2 points for each no answer and add 2 points for each yes answer to questions 11–20.

Scores	Grade	Interpretation
Below 60 =	F	This relationship is doomed to fail. You're in a codependent relationship with your electronics. They've become a choke collar, probably raising your stress and causing you to miss some of life's important moments.
60–69 =	D	Your electronic devices are masterminding you, possibly creating more stress than they're relieving.
70–79 =	C	You ping-pong between being in charge of your devices and caving to them. Becoming a stronger manager might free you up and help you de-stress.
80–89 =	B	You're doing a good job of showing your devices who's boss. You have more private time than electronic interference. Keep at it.
90–100 =	A	You're doing an excellent job of managing the line between electronic intrusion and focusing on other areas of your life.

What is Your Stress Age? (from Chapter 4)

Calculate your stress age by answering yes or no to the following questions, and then see what you can do about it.

___1. Do you make time just for yourself and nobody else?

___2. Are you easy on yourself when you make mistakes?

___3. Are you usually patient when you have to wait or stand in line?

___4. Do you live mostly in the present rather than worrying about the future?

___5. Do you treat yourself positively with kindness and respect?

___6. Do you get ample rest and exercise?

___7. Can you relax and have a good time without always being on the go?

___8. Are you good at saying no when you're overloaded and someone asks you to do something?

___9. Are you more happy-go-lucky than serious?

___10. Do you usually stay calm, cool and collected when things fall apart or don't go your way?

___11. Is your life usually overscheduled, inflexible, and rushed?

___12. Does it bother you when you're not in control of a situation?

___13. Are you frequently overwhelmed by everything on your plate?

___14. Do you frequently eat junk food or grab a bite on the run?

___15. Do you worry a lot while driving, falling asleep, or talking to others?

___16. Do you get upset when people don't meet your high standards?

___17. Do you often have a short fuse?

___18. Do little things set you off?

___19. Do you feel tired much of the time?

___20. Do you seek approval through people pleasing?

How to Calculate Your Stress Age

To compute your stress age, start with your actual age. Then for questions 1 through 10, subtract a year for each yes answer and add a year for each no answer. For questions 11 through 20, subtract a year for each no answer and add a year for each yes answer. The result is your stress age.

Are You Steel, Plastic, or Glass? (from Chapter 5)

Answer yes or no to each of the following questions:

___1. Do you seek approval from others through people pleasing?

___2. Do you judge yourself harshly?

___3. Do you resist change?

___4. Would you trade your life for someone else's?

___5. Do you spend a lot of time getting upset or angry over things you can't control?

___6. Are you afraid to let other people close to you?

___7. Do you waffle or fold under pressure?

___8. Do you feel that you're not enough and need someone or something to be complete?

___9. Do you usually put your needs behind those of others?

___10. Do you question your ability to do things?

___11. Do you feel worthy of other people's love?

___12. Do you believe you can turn a bad situation into a good one most of the time?

___13. Do you look on the bright side instead of the dark side in most situations?

___14. Do you enjoy your own company?

___15. Are you open to new ideas or different ways of doing things?

___16. Do you expect the best out of most situations?

___17. Do you believe in yourself?

___18. Do you tend to praise yourself or give yourself pep talks?

___19. Is it easy for you to express your true feelings?

___20. Are you open-minded?

How to Calculate Your Score

To compute your score, start with 60 points. Then subtract 2 points for each yes answer and add 2 points for each no answer to questions 1 through 10. Next, subtract 2 points for each no answer and add 2 points for each yes answer to questions 11 through 20. The higher your score the more stress hardy you are.

If your score is:

90–100: You're steel, and stress bounces off you.

70–89: You're plastic with some stress dents but also with some stress-hardy traits to build on.

Below 69: You're glass, at risk of being shattered by stress.

Are You a Mindful Marvel or a Mindless Menace? (from Chapter 12)

To get a sense of how mindful you are, answer yes or no to the following questions:

___1. Do you crack the whip, driving yourself with stress and worry?

___2. Is it hard for you to get stressful thoughts off your mind when you try to relax?

___3. Do you berate and punish yourself when you fall behind schedule?

___4. Does preoccupation with stress ever interfere with your personal relationships?

___5. Are you more task-focused than self-focused as you move through your day?

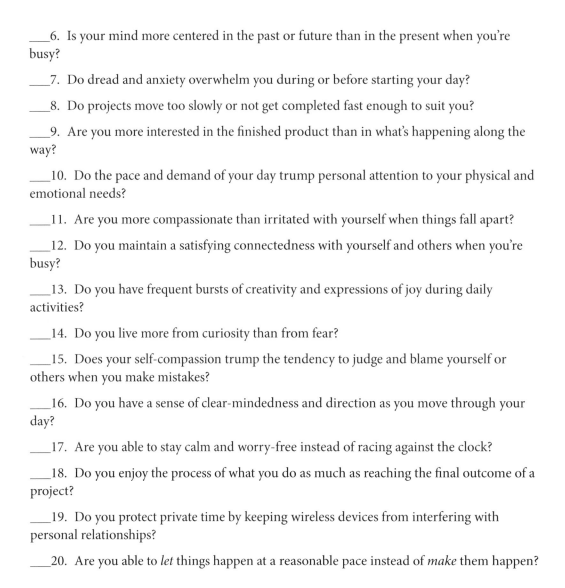

___6. Is your mind more centered in the past or future than in the present when you're busy?

___7. Do dread and anxiety overwhelm you during or before starting your day?

___8. Do projects move too slowly or not get completed fast enough to suit you?

___9. Are you more interested in the finished product than in what's happening along the way?

___10. Do the pace and demand of your day trump personal attention to your physical and emotional needs?

___11. Are you more compassionate than irritated with yourself when things fall apart?

___12. Do you maintain a satisfying connectedness with yourself and others when you're busy?

___13. Do you have frequent bursts of creativity and expressions of joy during daily activities?

___14. Do you live more from curiosity than from fear?

___15. Does your self-compassion trump the tendency to judge and blame yourself or others when you make mistakes?

___16. Do you have a sense of clear-mindedness and direction as you move through your day?

___17. Are you able to stay calm and worry-free instead of racing against the clock?

___18. Do you enjoy the process of what you do as much as reaching the final outcome of a project?

___19. Do you protect private time by keeping wireless devices from interfering with personal relationships?

___20. Are you able to *let* things happen at a reasonable pace instead of *make* them happen?

How to Calculate Your Score

To calculate your score, start with 60 points. Subtract 2 points for each yes answer to questions 1–10. Add 2 points for each no answer to questions 1–10. Subtract 2 points for each no answer to questions 11–20. Add 2 points for each yes answer to questions 11–20.

Scores	Grade	Interpretation
Below 60 =	F Poor	You're a mindless menace. Ask yourself if stress has eclipsed personal needs, causing you to lose touch with yourself and miss out on life's important moments.
60-69 =	D Below Average	You're more of a mindless menace than a mindful marvel. Stress has the upper hand and personal awareness and self-care are off the radar screen.
70-79 =	C Average	You're halfway between a mindless menace and a mindful marvel.
80-89 =	B Good	You're more of a mindful marvel than a mindless menace. You have some awareness of personal needs and probably come up for air or take breathers from time to time.
90-100 =	A Excellent	You're a mindful marvel. You're doing a great job of paying attention to your physical and emotional needs and treating yourself with loving kindness while meeting life's demands.

Is Your Job Hazardous to Your Health? (from Chapter 18)

Grade your workplace by answering yes or no to the following questions:

____1. Is your job fast-paced with little time to casually talk with coworkers?

____2. Does your work environment feel cold, sterile, and void of human touch?

____3. Does your workplace thrive on crisis, chaos, and pressure?

____4. Do you work for a company that emphasizes production and profit above the welfare and morale of its employees?

____5. Does success in your company hinge on putting in overtime on weekdays, weekends, and holidays?

____6. Do you think your company fosters workaholism?

____7. Are you constantly in a hurry, racing against the clock on your job?

____8. Have you had any stress-related illnesses caused by your job?

____9. Is it necessary to juggle many activities or projects to keep your head above water in your job?

____10. Does your company put you under the gun with short notice of high-pressured deadlines?

___11. Do you work for a company that puts the welfare of its employees above profit and production?

___12. Does your company have a caring attitude that shows concern for family, personal time, or stress reduction?

___13. Is your workplace relaxing, even paced, warm, and friendly?

___14. Does your job allow you to limit the amount of work you bring home and to reserve weekends and holidays for yourself and loved ones?

___15. Do you think your company has a long-term, vested interest in you as a human being versus a short-term interest?

___16. Does your company promote birthdays, holidays, socializing, or other celebrations as an integral part of your work schedule?

___17. Do you feel like a human being more often than a commodity in your job?

___18. Do you work with colleagues who are cooperative and supportive and with whom you can communicate?

___19. If you have a problem in your job, can you talk with supportive personnel who will listen and offer advice?

___20. Does your job give you any personal satisfaction, meaning, or purpose?

How to Calculate Your Score

To determine your job's report card, start with 60 points. Subtract 2 points for each yes answer to questions 1–10. Add 2 points for each no answer to questions 1–10. Subtract 2 points for each no answer to questions 11–20. Add 2 points for each yes answer to questions 11–20.

Scores	Grade	Interpretation
Below 60 =	F Poor	Consider a healthier workplace. You may already have the signs of stress and burnout or other physical symptoms that lead to bad health.
60–69 =	D Below average	
70–79 =	C Average	
80–89 =	B Good	
90–100 =	A Excellent	Stay put. Sounds like you've hit the jackpot of a low-stress, healthy work environment.

Are You a Careaholic? (from Chapter 19)

Take the following quiz to see if your caring patterns could be a way to relieve your own stress by using something outside yourself to fix something inside yourself.

Read the following statements and rate yourself according to how much each one pertains to you: When you finish, add the numbers in the blanks for your total score. 1 = never true, 2 = sometimes true, 3 = often true, 4 = always true.

____1. I get overly involved by taking on other people's problems.

____2. I feel overly responsible when bad things happen and feel that it's my role to make them better.

____3. I over-identify with others by feeling their emotions as if they are my own.

____4. I have an ongoing urge to take care of other people.

____5. I neglect my own needs in favor of caring for the needs of others.

____6. I take life too seriously and find it hard to play and have fun.

____7. I have a need to solve people's problems for them.

____8. I have not dealt with a lot of my own problems and stressors.

____9. I feel unworthy of love.

____10. I don't seem to have enough time for myself.

____11. I criticize myself too much.

____12. I'm afraid of being abandoned by those I love.

____13. My life seems to be in constant crisis.

____14. I don't feel good about myself unless I'm doing something for someone else.

____15. I don't know what to do with myself if I'm not helping someone.

____16. Whatever I do for someone doesn't seem to be enough.

____17. I have dedicated my life to helping others.

____18. I get a high from helping people with their problems.

____19. I have a need to take charge of most situations.

____20. I spend more time caretaking than I do socializing with friends or relaxing and having a good time.

____21. It's hard for me to relax when I'm not helping someone.

____22. I sometimes suffer excessive fatigue and compassion burnout.

____23. It's hard for me to keep emotional boundaries by saying no when someone wants to tell me their problems.

____24. I have developed health or physical problems from the stress of helping others or from excessive worry over someone else's problems.

____25. I seek approval through pleasing people and overcommitting myself.

How to Interpret Your Score

The higher your score, the more you lean toward careaholism. Use the following key to interpret your score:

25–49: You're not a careaholic

50–69: You're leaning toward careaholism

70–100: You're a careaholic

Risky Business: How to Spot a Workaholic (from Chapters 20 and 21)

Rate your boss, spouse, best friend, or yourself on the following work habits using the scale of 1: never true, 2: sometimes true, 3: often true, or 4: always true. Put the number that best describes the person you're rating in the blank beside the statement. Then add the numbers for your total score.

____1. I prefer to do most things instead of ask for help.

____2. I get impatient when I have to wait for someone else or when something takes too long.

____3. I seem to be in a hurry, racing against the clock.

____4. I get irritated when I'm interrupted while I'm in the middle of something.

____5. I stay busy with many irons in the fire.

____6. I engage in two or three activities at once such as eating lunch, working online, and talking on the phone.

____7. I overcommit myself by biting off more than I can chew.

____8. I feel guilty when I'm not working on something.

____9. It's important that I see the concrete results of my work.

____10. I'm more interested in the final result of my work than in the process.

____11. Things don't move fast enough or get done fast enough at work to suit me.

____12. I lose my temper when things don't go my way or work out to suit me.

____13. I ask the same question over again without realizing it after I've already been given the answer.

____14. I work in my head and think about future projects while tuning out the here and now

____15. I continue working after my coworkers have called it quits.

____16. I get angry when people don't meet my standards of perfection on the job.

____17. I get upset at work when I'm not in control.

____18. I tend to put myself under pressure from self-imposed work deadlines.

____19. It's hard for me to relax when I'm not working.

____20. I spend more time working than socializing with friends or enjoying hobbies or leisure activities.

____21. I dive into projects to get a head start before plans have been finalized.

____22. I get upset with myself for making even the smallest mistake on the job.

____23. I put more thought, time, and energy into work than into relationships with loved ones and friends.

____24. I forget, ignore, or minimize celebrations such as birthdays, reunions, anniversaries, or holidays.

____25. I make important job decisions before getting all the facts and thinking them through.

Interpreting Your Score

Now that you've added up your score, read on to find out how to interpret it.

25–56: Green light. You're a hard worker with good work-life balance whose work style isn't stressful for you or others.

57–66: Yellow light. You have a tendency to become busy and work to the exclusion of what's important to you. Your work habits are mildly stressful, but with modifications you can find balance and prevent job burnout.

67–100: Red light. You're chained to the desk and at risk for burnout. You have a double-barrel stress level, and other people get a busy signal when they try to connect with you.

APPENDIX B

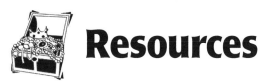

Resources

In this appendix, you'll learn about resources for further information so that you can explore topics discussed in this book in more depth. Plus, you'll discover support organizations and websites as well as CDs and DVDs devoted to the topic of stress management.

Chapter 1: Face-to-Face with Stress as a Fact of Life

Books

Adams, Kathleen. *Journal to the Self*. New York: Warner Books, 1990. Shows the transformative power of journaling to help you manage stress, work through problems, and recover from grief.

Dowrick, Stephanie. *Creative Journal Writing*. New York: Penguin, 2009. Inspirational instructions, practical suggestions, and helpful hints with starter exercises to give steam to your journal writing.

Kabat-Zinn, Jon. *Full Catastrophe Living: Using the Wisdom of Your Body and Mind to Face Stress, Pain, and Illness*. New York: Bantam, 1990. Contains the stress reduction and relaxation program taught at the University of Massachusetts Medical Center that is based on ten years of clinical experience.

Loehr, Jim. *The Power of Story: Rewrite Your Destiny in Business and Life*. New York: Free Press, 2007. Examines the way we tell stories about ourselves to ourselves and the way we can change those stories to reduce stress and transform our lives.

Selye, Hans. *The Stress of Life*. New York: McGraw-Hill, 1978. The father of stress explains how to overcome the harmful effects of stress and how to use stress to your advantage.

Support Organizations and Websites

American Institute of Stress
www.stress.org
124 Park Avenue
Yonkers, NY 10703
Stress125@optonline.net

Established at the request of Hans Selye as a clearinghouse for information on all stress-related subjects, including a newsletter on the latest advances in stress research and relevant health issues.

Duke Integrative Medicine
www.dukeintegrativemedicine.org
3475 Erwin Road
Durham, NC 27705

Sponsors stress-reduction programs, helping people cope with medical problems, job or family-related stress, and anxiety and depression.

The Center for Mindfulness in Medicine, Health Care, and Society
www.umassmed.edu
55 Lake Avenue North
Worcester, MA 01655

A visionary force and global leader in mind-body medicine, which hosts Jon Kabat-Zinn's eight-week mindfulness-based stress reduction (MBSR) program, an intensive training that asks participants to draw on their inner resources and natural capacity to actively engage in caring for themselves and finding greater balance, ease, and peace of mind.

Penn Program for Stress Management (PPM)
www.pennmedicine.org/stress
3930 Chestnut Street, 6th Floor
Philadelphia, PA 19104

A program designed to help you manage stress through the meditation-based process of mindfulness.

Chapter 2: When Stress Hits Home

Books

Chodron, Pema. *When Things Fall Apart: Heart Advice for Difficult Times.* Boston: Shambhala, 1997. Provides ways to reduce stress and go on living when overcome by pain, fear, and anxiety. Also on CD from Shambhala audio programs: www.shambhala.com.

Kornfield, Jack. *A Lamp in the Darkness.* Boulder, CO: Sounds True, 2011. Shows you how to illuminate your path through difficult times.

Lenson, Barry. *Good Stress, Bad Stress.* New York: Avalon, 2002. How to use good stress to perform at your best.

Luskin, Fred, and Ken Pelletier. *Stress Free for Good.* San Francisco, CA: HarperCollins, 2005. Presents ten scientifically proven life skills for stress reduction, physical health and vitality, and happiness.

Nepo, Mark. *The Book of Awakening.* San Francisco, CA: Conari Press, 2000. Reflections on having the life you want by being present in the life you have.

Singer, Thea. *Stress Less.* New York: Hudson Street Press, 2010. The new science that shows women how to rejuvenate the body and the mind.

Support Organizations and Websites

American Psychological Association
www.apa.org.publicinfo
750 First Street NE
Washington, DC 20002-4242

Provides research and facts to the public about stress and stress management.

Yale Stress Center
www.yalestress.org
2 Church Street South
Suite 209
New Haven, CT 06519

Offers education and services for decreasing the harmful impact of stress on health and improving your ability to regulate stress.

Chapter 3: Coping with Twenty-First Century Stress

Books

His Holiness the Dalai Lama, and Howard Cutler. *The Art of Happiness.* New York: Riverhead Books, 1998. Shows you how the power of an internal life strengthens you enough to navigate the stress the external world brings you.

Kundtz, David. *Quiet Mind: One-minute Retreats from a Busy World.* San Francisco, CA: Conari Press, 2000. A book of meditations and reflections to restore calm and clarity that hectic schedules steal from you.

LeClaire, Anne. *Listening Below the Noise: A Meditation on the Practice of Silence.* San Francisco, CA: HarperCollins, 2009. By detaching yourself from the hustle of your hectic lifestyle, you can listen to your deepest self and find a center from which to live.

Loehr, Jim, and Tony Schwartz. *The Power of Full Engagement: Managing Energy, Not Time, Is the Key to High Performance and Personal Renewal.* New York: Free Press, 2003. Shows you how to maximize the use of the fixed number of hours in your day.

Robinson, Bryan, and Nancy Chase. *High-Performing Families: Causes, Consequences, and Clinical Solutions.* Washington, DC: American Counseling Association, 2001. A look at families on the fast track—what causes it, what the consequences are, and what solutions are possible.

Robinson, Joe *The Guide to Getting a life.* Berkeley, CA: Berkeley Publications Group, 2003. An impassioned manifesto about the need to take vacations for restoration of body and soul.

Chapter 4: Preventing Burnout and Creating a Stress-Free Life

Books

Figley, Charles. *Treating Compassion Fatigue.* New York: Brunner-Routledge, 2002. A thorough examination addressing the burnout that comes from caregiving and the treatment that is available.

Support Organizations and Websites

American Counseling Association
www.counseling.org
5999 Stevenson Avenue
Alexandria, VA 22304

Promotes the counseling profession and those served through work in advocacy, research, and professional standards, including publications on stress and burnout.

International Stress Management Association
www.isma.org.uk/
PO Box 491
Bradley Stoke, Bristol BS34 9AH

Educates the public in the field of well-being and stress prevention worldwide through sound knowledge and practice in stress reduction.

WebMD
www.webmd.com

Provides valuable resources on stress-related topics and other mental health issues related to stress, burnout, and prevention.

Audiovisual

Online program: Bob Stahl and Elisha Goldstein. *Mindfulness, Anxiety and Stress Program.* A self-directed, multimedia program. Go to www.liveworld.com/shops/mh1/mindfulness-anxiety-and-stress.aspx.

Chapter 5: Mastering a Stress-Hardy Coping Style

Books

Aron, Elaine. *The Highly Sensitive Person.* New York: Broadway Books, 1996. How to thrive when the world overwhelms you.

Hallowell, Edward. *Worry: Controlling it and using it Wisely.* New York: Pantheon, 1997. A guidebook to help you understand and deal with the underlying causes of unnecessary worry.

Leahey, Robert. *The Worry Cure: Seven Steps to Stop Worry from Stopping You.* New York: Three Rivers Press, 2005. A guide to help you understand and show you how to handle worry about relationships, money, health, and work.

Reivich, Karen, and Andrew Shatte. *The Resilience Factor: Seven Keys to Finding Your Inner Strength and Overcoming Life's Hurdles.* New York: Broadway Books, 2002. How changing the way you think will change the stress in your life for good.

Support Organizations and Websites

The Trauma Resource Institute

www.traumaresourceinstitute.com
PO Box 1891
Claremont, CA 91711

Holds the mission of restoring resiliency after trauma by expanding bottom-up capacity, taking people from despair to hope.

The National Institute of Mental Health

www.nimh.nih.gov
6001 Executive Blvd.
Room 8184, MSG 9663
Bethesda, MD 20892-9663
Nimhinfo@nih.gov

Serves to transform the understanding and treatment of mental illness through research and dissemination of information on stress and anxiety.

Audiovisuals

Naparstek, Bellerath. *Mind-Body Exercises for Stress-Hardiness Optimization*. Solon, Ohio: Playaway, 2010, CD.

Chapter 6: The Savvy Remedy for Stressful Eating Habits

Books

Altman, Donald. *Meal by Meal*. Novato, CA: New World Library, 2004. Includes 365 daily meditations for finding balance through mindful eating.

Chozen, Jan. *Mindful Eating*. Boston: Shambhala Publishers, 2009. Techniques for rediscovering a healthy and joyful relationship with food by eating mindfully.

Ornish, Dean. *Stress, Diet, and Your Heart*. New York: Signet Books, 1982. A lifetime program for healing your heart without drugs or surgery.

Thich Nhất Hanh, and Lilian Cheung. *Savor: Mindful Eating, Mindful Life*. New York: Harperone, 2010. Helps you achieve a healthy weight and well-being through good nutrition and sound eating habits.

Wansink, Brian. *Mindless Eating: Why We Eat More Than We Think*. New York: Bantam, 2010. Explores why we eat mindlessly for comfort and provides tips on how you can eat more mindfully and still de-stress.

Weil, Andrew. *Eating Well for Optimum Health*. New York: Knopf, 2000. An essential guide to bringing health and pleasure back to eating.

Support Organizations and Websites

National Eating Disorders Association
www.nationaleatingdisorders.org
603 Stewart Street, Suite 803
Seattle, WA 98101

Dedicated to providing help and hope to those affected by eating disorders.

Audiovisuals

Weil, Andrew. *Eating Well for Optimum Health*. Random House Audio, 2006, DVD.

Chapter 7: Exercise is Good Stress Medicine

Books

Agus, David. *The End of Illness*. New York: The Free Press, 2011. A systemic perspective on health that allows you to live a long, fulfilling, disease-free life.

Oswald, Christopher, and Stanley Bacso. *Stretching for Fitness, Health, and Performance: The Complete Handbook for All Ages and Fitness Levels*. New York: Sterling Publications, 2003. Explicit stretch-by-stretch photos showing you the health benefits of stretching along with stretching routines for office, car, and plane for children to senior citizens.

Roizen, Michael, and Mehmet Oz. *YOU: The Owner's Manual*. New York: Harpercollins, 2005. An insider's guide to the body that will make you healthier and younger.

Runyon, Chuck, and Brian Zehetner, and Rebecca DeRossett. *Working Out Sucks*. Boston, MA: DaCapo Press, 2012. The only twenty-one day kick-start plan for total health and fitness that helps you rethink unhealthy habits, destructive attitudes, and misinformation about health.

Support Organizations and Websites

American Academy of Podiatric Sports Medicine
www.aapsm.org
109 Greenwich Drive
Walkersville, MD 21793

Serves to advance the understanding, prevention, and management of lower extremity and fitness injuries to the public.

American Council on Exercise
www.acefitness.org

A nonprofit fitness certification and education provider committed to enriching quality of life through safe and effective physical activity.

4851 Paramount Drive
San Diego, CA 92123

Chapter 8: Rx for Your Daily Doses of Sleep

Books

Edlund, Matthew. *The Power of Rest: Why Sleep Alone is Not Enough.* New York: HarperCollins, 2010. Strategies for relaxed concentration to help you become more alert and fully engaged with your body, your work, and the people you love.

Weil, Andrew. *Healthy Aging: A Lifelong Guide to Your Well-Being.* New York: Anchor, 2007. How to age gracefully from stress to sex to rest and sleep.

Support Organizations and Websites

American Academy of Sleep Medicine
www.aasmnet.org
2510 North Frontage Road
Darien, IL 60561

Sleep Medicine Association for professionals dedicated to the treatment of sleep disorders such as sleep apnea and insomnia.

Better Sleep Council
www.bettersleep.org
501 Wythe Street
Alexandria, VA 22314-1917

Promotes the importance of sleep to good health and quality of life and the value of a healthy sleep environment in pursuit of a good night's sleep.

National Sleep Foundation
www.sleepfoundation.org
1010 North Glebe Road, Suite 310
Arlington, VA 22201

Supports public education, sleep related research, and advocacy related to sleep disorders and sleep deprivation.

Audiovisuals

Stahl, Bob. *Working with Insomnia and Sleep Challenges*. Bob Stahl, 2005, CD.

Chapter 9: Stress-Proofing Your Brain

Books

Amen, Daniel. *Change Your Brain, Change Your Body*. New York: Three Rivers Press, 2010. How to use your brain to get and keep the body you want.

Begley, Sharon. *Train Your Mind, Change Your Brain*. New York: Ballantine, 2008. How science reveals your extraordinary potential to transform yourself by training your mind.

Doidge, Norman. *The Brain that Changes Itself*. New York: Penguin, 2007. Stories of personal triumph, showing how you can change and stress-proof your pliable brain.

Hanson, Rick, and Richard Mendius. *Buddha's Brain: The Practical Neuroscience of Happiness, Love and Wisdom*. Oakland, CA: New Harbinger Publications, 2009. Draws on the latest research in neuroscience on how you can stimulate and strengthen your brain for a less stressful, more fulfilling life.

Hanson, Rick. *Just One Thing: Developing a Buddha Brain One Simple Practice at a Time*. Oakland, CA: New Harbinger, 2011. Offers simple brain training practices you can do every day to protect against stress.

Newberg, Andrew, and Mark Waldman. *How GOD Changes Your Brain*. New York: Ballantine Books, 2010. Breakthrough findings in neuroscience showing the link between brain chemistry, spirituality, and stress reduction.

Rossman, Martin. *The Worry Solution: Using Breakthrough Brain Science to Turn Stress and Anxiety into Confidence and Happiness*. New York: Crown, 2010. An easy-to-follow plan to relieve stress and anxiety by training your brain's imagination.

Schwartz, Jeffrey, and Sharon Begley. T*he Mind and the Brain: Neuroplasticity and the Power of Mental Force*. New York: HarperCollins, 2002. How you can make your own neural pathways by focusing your attention away from negativity and toward positivity.

Siegel, Daniel. *The Mindful Brain*. New York: Norton, 2007. How mindfulness promotes resonance circuits in the brain that allow you to attune to your internal life and that of others.

Support Organizations and Websites

The Wellspring Institute. www.wisebrain.org. 25 Mitchell Boulevard, Suite. San Rafael, CA 94903

Audiovisuals

Hanson, Rick. *Stress-Proof Your Brain*. Boulder, CO: Sounds True, Inc., 2010, CD. Two CDs of information and practices to rewire neural pathways for stress relief.

Rossman, Martin. The Worry Solution. Audio CD. Order from: Amazon.com

Provides resources for changing the brain for the better--for more happiness, love, and wisdom. Publishes The Wise Brain Bulletin.

Chapter 10: Relaxing Your Body and Physical Wellness

Books

Cope, Stephen. *Yoga and the Quest for the True Self*. New York: Bantam, 2000. The use of yoga as a communion between Western psychotherapy and Eastern yogic philosophy for those in search of stress relief.

Crawford, Jacqueline, Karen Pomerinke, and Donald Smith. *Therapy Pets: The Animal-Human Healing Partnership*. Amherst, NY: Prometheus Books, 2003. Shows how the field of animal-assisted therapy is having remarkable success training animals to reduce stress and enhance the lives of people with medical problems.

Levine, Peter. *Waking the Tiger: Healing Trauma*. Berkeley, CA: North Atlantic Books, 1997. A series of exercises help you focus on body sensations to heal trauma and reduce stress.

McKay, Matthew, and Patrick Fanning. *The Relaxation and Stress Reduction Workbook*.

Oakland, CA: New Harbinger, 1997. Brings together tension-relieving exercises for a stress-free body.

Robbins, Jim. *A Symphony in the Brain*. New York: Grove Press, 2008. The evolution of the new brain wave biofeedback.

Scaer, Robert. *The Body Bears the Burden: Trauma, Dissociation and Disease*. Binghamton, NY: Haworth Press, 2001. Provides the latest strategies to deal with stress and minimize emotional and physical damage.

Weintraub, Amy. *Yoga for Depression*. New York: Broadway Books, 2004. A compassionate guide to relieving suffering through yoga.

Support Organizations and Websites

American Massage Therapy Association
www.amtamassage.org

Provides an online directory of massage therapists in the United States. Find a certified massage therapist at: www.findamassagetherapist.org

The EEG Directory
www.eegdirectory.com

A searchable database of neuro-feedback providers around the world.

Magazines

Yoga Journal

www.yogajournal.com

Chapter 11: Calming Your Mind and Restorative Rest

Books

Ackerman, Diane. *Deep Play*. New York: Vintage Books, 2000. The exalted state of transcendence through emotionally and physically vigorous activities.

Benson, Herbert. *The Relaxation Response*. New York: HarperCollins, 2000. Shows how to use the relaxation response to relieve the tension of modern-day stress.

Benson, Herbert, and William Proctor. *Relaxation Revolution*. New York: Scribner, 2010. The latest scientific proof that your mind can heal your body with descriptions of how to apply mind-body techniques to treat a variety of health conditions.

Brantley, Jeffrey, and Wendy Millstine. *Daily Meditations for Calming Your Anxious Mind*. Oakland, CA: New Harbinger Publications, 2008. Provides sixty-four meditations and visualizations on how to leave stress and worry behind and attune to the present moment in an attentive, nonjudgmental way.

Gawain, Shakti. *Creative Visualization: Use the Power of Your Imagination to Create What You Want in Your Life*. Novato, CA: New World Library, 2002. Describes the art of using mental imagery and affirmation to produce positive changes in your life.

Merton, Thomas. *New Seeds of Contemplation*. New York: New Direction Books, 2007. Seeks to awaken the dormant inner depths of the spirit with contemplation.

Moore, Thomas. *Care of the Soul*. New York: Harper Collins, 1994. A guide for cultivating depth and sacredness in everyday life.

Tolle, Eckhart. *Stillness Speaks*. Novato, CA: New World Library, 2003. How to connect to the stillness that brings you inner peace.

Support Organizations and Websites

The Benson-Henry Institute for Mind/Body Medicine
www.massgeneral.org
Massachusetts General Hospital
55 Fruit Street
Boston, MA 02114

A mind/body website that offers help if you're experiencing the negative effects of stress: steps for how to elicit the relaxation response and a line of CDs for relaxation.

Audiovisuals

Silverlake Music
www.silverlakemusic.com

CDs and DVDs for relaxation, meditation, yoga, sleep, and massage.

Chapter 12: Mindful Awareness and Stress Reduction

Books

Boorstein, Sylvia. *Don't Just Do Something, Sit There: A Mindfulness Retreat with Sylvia*

Boorstein. San Francisco, CA: Harper, 1996. A lively and down-to-earth guide to your own three-day mindfulness meditation retreat.

Boorstein, Sylvia. *Happiness is an Inside Job.* New York: Random House, 2008. Shows how the practice of mindfulness and loving kindness quiets your mind, deepens concentration, and reduces stress. Also available on CD.

Lipsenthal, Lee. *Enjoy Every Sandwich.* New York: Crown, 2011. An inspirational book on living a fearless, full life as if each day were your last.

Kabat-Zinn, Jon. *Wherever You Go, There You Are: Mindfulness Meditation in Everyday Life.* New York: Hyperion, 1994. Provides access to the essence of meditation and its applications for beginners and those who want to deepen their practice.

Siegel, Ronald. *The Mindful Solution: Everyday Practices for Everyday Problems.* New York: Guilford Press, 2010. Offers a path to well-being and comprehensive mindfulness practices for coping with life's inevitable hurdles.

Smalley, Susan, and Diana Winston. *Fully Present: The Science, Art, and Practice of Mindfulness.* Philadelphia, PA: DaCapo Press, 2010. Gives a scientific explanation of how mindfulness puts the brakes on stress, complete with research on how your brain responds to meditation and practical tips and exercises for practice.

Thich Nhat Hanh. *Walking Meditation.* Boulder Co: Sounds True, 2006. A book detailing the various kinds of walking meditations and how to do them along with DVD and CD.

Tolle, Eckhart. *The Power of Now: A Guide to Spiritual Enlightenment.* Novato, CA: New World Library, 2004. A spiritual approach to inner peace that brings tranquility by leaving the analytical mind and its false created self, the ego, behind.

Audiovisuals

eMindful
www.eMindful.com

A global Internet source for comprehensive health and wellness services with online classes and an interactive blog.

Mindfulness Meditation Practice CDs and Tapes
www.mindfulnesstapes.com

A website dedicated to making available high-quality stress reduction CDs and tapes by Dr. Jon Kabat-Zinn to help you develop and deepen your personal meditation practice.

Thich Nhat Hanh. *The Art of Mindful Living: How to Bring Love, Compassion, and Inner Peace into Your Daily Life.* Boulder, CO: Sounds True, 2000, CD.

Thich Nhat Hanh. *The Present Moment.* Boulder, CO: Sounds True, 2003, CD. A retreat on the practice of mindfulness

Thich Nhat Hanh. *Living Without Stress or Fear. Boulder, CO:* Sounds True, 2009, CD.

Chapter 13: Meditation Practices and Stress Resilience

Books

Kornfield, Jack. *A Path with Heart.* New York: Bantam, 2002. A Guide through the perils and promises of spiritual life.

Kornfield, Jack. *Meditation for Beginners.* Boulder, CO: Sounds True Publishers, 2008. The benefits of meditation, how to get started, go deeper, and maintain a daily practice.

Kornfield, Jack. *The Buddha is Still Teaching.* Boston: Shambhala, 2010. Selections from the most highly regarded Buddhist teachers of the twenty-first century.

Salzberg, Sharon, and Joseph Goldstein. *Insight Meditation.* Boulder, CO: Sounds True, 2001. A workbook, a set of informational cards, and two CDs that takes you step-by-step through a comprehensive training course in basic meditation.

Thich Nhat Hanh. *Peace is Every Step: The Path of Mindfulness in Everyday Life.* New York: Bantam, 1991. Brings ancient Buddhist teachings to modern problems.

Support Organizations and Websites

Buddhist Information and Education Network
www.buddhanet.net
Bodhi Tree Forest Monastery & Retreat Centre
78 Bentley Road, Tullera, via Lismore
NSW 2480 Australia

A network of Buddhist information and education, including information on Buddhist studies worldwide, a world Buddhist directory, online magazine, and book library and library resources.

Esalen Institute
www.esalen.org
55000 Highway 1
Big Sur, CA 93920

An education center located on the Big Sur coastline, Esalen hosts a convergence of mountains and sea, mind and body, East and West, and meditation and action through workshops on meditation, yoga, movement, work-study programs, and personal retreats to nourish your body, mind, and heart.

Insight Meditation Society
www.dharma.org/ims
1230 Pleasant Street
Barre, MA 01005

One of the Western world's most respected retreat centers for learning and deepening your meditation practices.

Institute for Meditation and Psychotherapy
www.meditationandpsychotherapy.org
35 Pleasant Street
Newton, MA 02459

Dedicated to the training of mental health professionals interested in the integration of mindfulness, meditation, and psychotherapy.

Kripalu Center for Yoga and Health
www.kripalu.org
PO Box 309
Stockbridge, MA 01262

Offers workshops and retreats, a professional school, and online newsletter—all designed to teach the art and science of yoga and to produce thriving and healthy individuals and society.

Omega Institute
Rhinebeck, NY
www.eomega.org
150 Lake Drive
Rhinebeck, NY 12572

Omega retreats are designed to help you unplug from life's demands and deal with the daily pressures through de-stressing, relaxing, and renewing your soul. The center offers workshops, trainings, retreats, and vacations, where you can create your own schedule of meditation, massage, bodywork, acupuncture, tai chi, qigong, and physical activities.

Audiovisuals

Goldstein, Joseph, and Sharon Salzberg. *Insight Meditation: An In-Depth Correspondence Course.* Boulder, CO: Sounds True, 2004, CD.

Kornfield, Jack. *Meditation for Beginners.* Boulder, CO: Sounds True, 2008, CD.

Kornfield, Jack. *The Inner Art of Meditation.* Boulder, CO: Sounds True, 2004, CD.

Stahl, Bob. *Body Scan and Sitting Meditation.*
[Order from: www.mindfulnessprograms.com.]

Stahl, Bob. *Mindful Qigong and Loving-Kindness Meditation.*
[DVD. Order from: www.mindfulnessprograms.com]

Chapter 14: Stress-Buffering Your Mind's Negativity

Books

Brach, Tara. *Radical Acceptance: Embracing Your Life with the Heart of a Buddha.* New York: Bantam, 2003. Helps you realize your true nature and gain self-acceptance.

Cameron, Julia. *The Artist's Way: A Spiritual Path to Higher Creativity*. New York: Tarcher, 2002. Discusses your enemy within—core negative beliefs—and shows the power of affirmations as your biggest ally in achieving inner peace.

Gilbert, Paul. *The Compassionate Mind: A New Approach to Life's Challenges.* Oakland, CA: New Harbinger Publications, 2009. Reveals the evolutionary and social reasons why the brain reacts so readily to threats and shows we are also wired for kindness and compassion.

Goleman, Daniel. *Destructive Emotions: How Can We Overcome Them?* New York: Bantam, 2003. A dialogue between His Holiness the Dalai Lama, Western scholars, Buddhist scholars, neuroscientists, and philosophers on how to overcome negativity. Also available on CD.

Kundtz, David. *Awakened Mind.* San Francisco, CA: Conari Press, 2009. One-minute wake-up calls to a bold and mindful life.

Love, Patricia, and Jon Carlson. *Never Be Lonely Again.* Deerfield Beach, FL: HCI Publications, 2011. The way out of emptiness, isolation, and a life unfulfilled.

Siegel, Daniel. *Mindsight: The New Science of Personal Transformation.* New York: Bantam,

2010. Shows you how to make positive changes in your brain and your life and heal from stressful events.

Williams, Mark, John Teasdale, Zindel Segal, and Jon Kabat-Zinn. *The Mindful Way Through Depression.* New York: Guilford, 2007. Walks you through an avenue out of depression.

Support Organizations and Websites

Mind and Life Institute
7007 Winchester Circle, Suite 100
Boulder, CO 80301
www.mindandlife.org

Seeks to understand the human mind and build a scientific understanding of how to cultivate compassion and wisdom. Website contains an interactive mind and life blog.

Audiovisuals

Chodron, Pema. *Don't Bite the Hook.* Boston: Shambhala, 2008, CD. Finding freedom from anger, resentment, and other destructive emotions.

Hanson, Rick. *Meditations to Change Your Brain.* Boulder, CO: Sounds True, 2009, CD. How to unwire negativity and tap the power of self-directed neuroplasticity.

Chapter 15: Outwitting Stress by Changing Your Thinking

Books

Beck, Judith. *Cognitive Behavior Therapy: Basics and Beyond.* New York: Guilford Press, 2011. A detailed and clear account of the basic principles of cognitive behavior therapy, one of the most common strategies for reframing your outlook, and managing stress.

Burns, David. *Feeling Good: The New Mood Therapy.* New York: HarperCollins, 1999. An outline of the scientifically tested cognitive techniques on how to change your perspective, lift your spirits, and develop a positive outlook on life.

Ellis, Albert. and Windy Dryden. *The Practice of Rational Emotive Behavior Therapy (2nd Ed.).* New York: Springer Publications, 2007. An academic guide describing the basic principles of rational emotive behavior therapy to help you change your self-defeating thoughts, feelings, and behaviors that can lead to stress and burnout.

Hayes, Steven, and Spencer Smith. *Get Out of Your Mind and into Your Life.* Oakland, CA: New Harbinger Publications, 2005. Gives you a different perspective on your problems and your life and the way you live it through acceptance and commitment therapy (ACT).

Richo, David. *The Five Things We Cannot Change . . . and the Happiness We find by Embracing Them.* Boston: Shambhala, 2006. A stress-reducing guide to help you come to accept life on its terms as it is and not as you want it to be.

Support Organizations and Websites

Beck Institute for Cognitive Therapy and Research
www.beckinstitute.org
GSB Building
City Line & Belmont Avenues
Suite 700
Bala Cynwyd, PA 19004-1610

Provides state-of-the-art psychotherapy and research opportunities and serves as an international training ground for cognitive therapists at all levels.

Chapter 16: Stress Relief with Positivity, Optimism, and Self-Compassion

Books

Beattie, Melody. *Gratitude.* Center City, MN: Hazelden, 2007. Features stirring affirmations inspiring readers to appreciate the really important things in life.

Chodron, Pema. *Awakening Loving-Kindness.* Boston: Shambhala, 1996. Provides teachings to help you remain wholeheartedly awake and stress resistant to everything in your life through the practice of loving-kindness.

Fredrickson, Barbara. *Positivity.* New York: Three Rivers Press, 2009. Top-notch research on how positive emotions can stress-proof you to see new possibilities, bounce back from setbacks, connect with others, and become the best version of yourself.

Germer, Christopher. *The Mindful Path to Self-Compassion.* New York: Guilford Publications, 2009. Shows you how through self-compassion you can free yourself from destructive thoughts and emotions.

Ladner, Lorne. *The Lost Art of Compassion.* San Francisco, CA: HarperCollins, 2004. Explores one of the most powerful inner resources—that of compassion—for managing stress and creating a life of happiness and contentment.

Neff, Kristin. *Self-Compassion.* New York: HarperCollins, 2011. A scientific and personal look at how self-compassion reduces stress and promotes stress resilience and happiness.

Salzberg, Sharon. *The Force of Kindness.* Boulder, CO: Sounds True, 2010. Instruction and exercises to help you discover the power of loving-kindness within you to guide your daily life.

Seligman, Martin. *Authentic Happiness.* New York: The Free Press, 2002. Using positivity to realize your potential for lasting fulfillment.

Support Organizations and Websites

Positive Emotions and Psychophysiology Laboratory
www.positiveemotions.org

Studies how people's positive emotions affect thinking patterns, social behavior, and physiological reactions. The ultimate goal is to understand how positive emotions can combat stress, create well-being, and transform lives for the better.

Self-Compassion: A Healthier Way of Relating to Yourself
www.self-compassion.org

Dr. Neff provides information about self-compassion; intended for students, researchers, and the general public. The site contains exercises to increase self-compassion, self-compassion meditations, and a test to gauge how self-compassionate you are.

Chapter 17: De-stressing Your Personal Surroundings

Books

Beattie, Melody. *The Language of Letting Go.* Center City, MN: Hazelden, 1990. Daily meditations on codependency. Also available on CD.

Cabarga, Leslie. *The Designer's Guide to Color Combinations.*Cincinatti, Ohio: North Light Books, 2003. Contains a large collection of color combinations that work together.

Walch, Margaret. *Living Colors: A Definitive Guide to Color Palettes Through the Ages.* San Francisco, CA: Chronicle Books, 1995. A spiral-bound workbook that shows eighty classic color schemes from art and design history.

Audiovisuals

CDs, DVDs, and MP3 downloads of nature sound recordings for relaxation, reflection, and meditation:

Listening Earth
www.listeningearth.com

Nature Guy
www.natureguystudio.com

Nature Sounds
www.naturesounds.ca

Nature Sounds
www.naturesounds.us

Real Nature Sounds
www.realnaturesounds.com

Serenity Supply
www.serenitysupply.com

Wild Sanctuary
www.wildsanctuary.com

Wildlife Sound Recording
www.wildlife-sound.org

Chapter 18: Sidestepping Work Stress and Job Burnout

Books

Carroll, Michael. *Awake at Work: 35 Practical Buddhist Principles for Discovering Clarity and Balance in the Midst of Work Chaos.* Boston: Shambahla Publishers, 2004. A Buddhist approach to transforming the common hassles and anxieties of the workplace into valuable opportunities.

Crowley, Katherine. *Working with you is Killing Me: Freeing Yourself from Emotional Traps at Work.* New York: Warner Books, 2006. Tips on extreme bosses, corporate culture, and how to protect yourself in the workplace.

Ferriss, Timothy. *The 4-Hour Workweek.* New York: Crown, 2009. Reconstructing your life so that it's not all about work.

His Holiness the Dalai Lama. *The Art of Happiness at Work.* New York: Riverhead Books, 2003. A series of conversations with His Holiness the Dalai Lama, recounted by psychiatrist Howard Cutler, discussing ways to turn work and careers into a satisfying and meaningful part of your life.

Schwartz, Tony. *The Way We're Working Isn't Working.* New York: Simon and Schuster, 2010. A blueprint for a new way of working and a more satisfying way of life, providing a roadmap to fueling a fully engaged workforce.

Sormaz, Heidi, and Bruce Tulgan. *Performance Under Pressure.* Amherst, MA: Rainmaker Thinking, 2003. Managing stress in the workplace.

Support Organizations and Websites

National Institute for Occupational Safety and Health (NIOSH)
www.cdc.gov/niosh
Center for Disease Control and Prevention
1600 Clifton Road
Atlanta, GA 30333

Provides national and world leadership to prevent workplace illnesses and injuries and conducts research into occupational safety and health matters.

Audiovisuals

Reskin, Ann, *Working with Stress.* Atlanta, GA: National Institute for Occupational Safety and Health, 2002. Video. An educational video program on workplace stress describing factors that create or worsen job stress, and practical measures to reduce them.

Goldstein, Elisha. *Mindful Solutions for Success and Stress Reduction at Work.* Los Angeles, CA: Mindful Solutions, 2010

Chapter 19: Stress-Resistant Relationships

Books

Chapman, Gary. *The 5 Love Languages: The Secret to Love That Lasts.* Chicago: Northfield Publishing, 2010. Describes five types of love languages that deepens communication and intimacy.

Gottman, John. *The Seven Principles for Making Marriage Work.* New York: Crown, 1999. Explores the signals of problem relationships and the steps for improving them.

Hendrix, Harville. *Getting the Love You Want: A Guide for Couples.* New York: Harper & Row, 1988. A look at how perceptual illusions from your past (called the imago) block your connectivity in relationships and how to overcome obstacles.

Heitler, Susan. *The Power of Two: Secrets to a Strong and Loving Marriage.* Oakland, CA: New Harbinger, 1997. Uses simple tools and guidelines to show how to develop strong communication and deepen intimacy.

Luskin, Fred. *Forgive for Good.* San Francisco, CA: HarperCollins, 2003. New insight into the healing powers and medical benefits of forgiveness.

Audiovisuals

Luskin, Fred. *The Nine Steps to Forgiveness.* Vero Beach, FL: eMindful publications, 2004, CD.

Support Organizations and Websites

American Association for Marriage and Family Therapy
www.aamft.org
112 South Alfred Street
Alexandria, VA 22314-3061

Offers resources for consumers on a wide range of problems, including marital strife and family stress, anxiety and depression, and parent-child conflict, plus a search engine for finding a qualified therapist nationwide.

Imago Relationships International
www.imagotherapy.com
160 Broadway
East Building, Suite 1001
New York, NY 10038

Offers face-to-face learning opportunities through workshops for couples and singles and products that teach the dynamics of the love relationship in achieving personal growth.

Chapter 20: Stress Management and Addictive Behaviors

Books

Armstrong, Karen. *Twelve Steps to a Compassionate Life.* New York: Knopf, 2010. Concrete ways to embrace self-compassion through a 12-Step framework.

Beattie, Melody. *Codependent No More.* Center City, MN: Hazelden, 1986. How to stop controlling others and start caring for yourself.

Bien, Thomas, and Beverly Bien. *Mindful Recovery: A Spiritual Path to Healing From Addiction.* New York: Wiley, 2002. Shows you how to use mindfulness to enjoy the present moment and recover from addiction.

Houlder, Dominic, and Kulananda Houlder. *Mindfulness and Money.* New York: Broadway Books, 2002. Lays out the path of abundance with practical wisdom, exercises, meditations, and real-life examples.

Support Organizations and Websites

Alcoholics Anonymous

www.aa.org

A fellowship of men and women who share their experience, strength, and hope to solve their common problems and help others to recover from alcoholism.

Codependents Anonymous

www.coda.org

A fellowship of men and women whose common purpose is to develop healthy relationships.

Debtors Anonymous

www.debtorsanonymous.org

A fellowship of men and women who share their experience, strength, and hope with each other so that they may solve their common problem and help others to recover from compulsively getting into debt.

Food Addicts Anonymous

www.foodaddictsanonymous.org

An organization that believes that food addiction is a biochemical disorder that occurs at a cellular level and therefore cannot be cured by willpower or by therapy alone. This 12-Step program believes that food addiction can be managed by abstaining (eliminating) from addictive foods, following a program of sound nutrition (a food plan), and working the 12-Steps of the program.

Gamblers Anonymous

www.gamblersanonymous.org

A fellowship of men and women who share their experience, strength, and hope with each other so that they may solve their common problem and help others recover from a gambling problem.

Narcotics Anonymous

www.na.org

A membership open to all drug addicts regardless of the particular drug or combination of drugs used. Members share their success and challenges in overcoming active addiction and living drug-free, productive lives through the principles contained within the 12 Steps.

National Council on Problem Gambling

www.ncpgambling.org

Committed to increasing public awareness of pathological gambling and to finding new ways to support gamblers in recovery.

Overeaters Anonymous

www.oa.org

A program of recovery from compulsive eating using the 12 Steps. Overeaters Anonymous is not just about weight loss, gain, maintenance, obesity or diets; it addresses physical, emotional, and spiritual well-being as well.

Sex Addicts Anonymous

www.sexaa.org

A fellowship of men and women who share their experience, strength, and hope with each other for the purpose of finding freedom from addictive sexual behavior and helping others recover from sex addiction. The organization offers an accepting, nonthreatening environment, where people can share their common struggles and apply the principles of the 12-Steps to their everyday lives.

Sexaholics Anonymous

www.sa.org

A fellowship of men and women who share their experience, strength, and hope with each other so that they may stay sexually sober and help others achieve sexual sobriety.

Sex and Love Addicts Anonymous

www.slaafws.org

A 12-Step fellowship of men and women who offer help to anyone who has a sex addiction or love addiction or both and wants to do something about it.

Spenders Anonymous
www.spenders.org

A 12-Step program based on the principles of Alcoholics Anonymous to get the word out to compulsive spenders who are still suffering. Their message is that you are not alone and that you too can find peace and serenity through the 12-Steps of Spenders Anonymous.

Workaholics Anonymous
www.workaholics-anonymous.org

A membership whose primary purpose is to help members stop working compulsively and to carry the message of recovery to workaholics who still suffer.

Audiovisuals

Goldstein, Elisha, and Stefanie Goldstein. *Mindful Solutions for Addiction and Relapse Prevention.* Los Angeles, CA: Mindful Solutions, 2010, CD.

Chapter 21: Maintaining Work-Life Balance and Stress Resilience

Books

Chodron, Pema. *The Places that Scare You.* Boston: Shambhala, 2005. A guide to fearlessness in difficult times. Also comes in CD.

Pierce, Gregory. *Spirituality at Work: 10 Ways to Balance Your Life on the Job.* New York: Loyola Press, 2005. How keep a spiritual even keel while working.

Robinson, Bryan. *Chained to the Desk: A Guidebook for Workaholics, Their Partners and Children, and the Clinicians Who Treat Them.* New York: New York University Press, 2007. Describes the workaholic struggle between the work life of *doing* and overdoing versus the personal life of *being* and how to de-stress and achieve work-life balance.

Robinson, Bryan. *The Art of Confident Living: Ten Practices for Taking Charge of Your Life.* Deerfield Beach, FL: Health Communications, 2009. Your guide to realizing how you're treating life and finding your stress-resilient self that resides in everyone.

Rubin, Gretchen. *The Happiness Project.* New York: HarperCollins, 2009. Shows how novelty and challenges are powerful sources of stress resilience and happiness.

Siebert, Al. *The Resiliency Advantage.* San Francisco, CA: Berrett-Koehler Publishers, 2005. Shows you how to become stress resilient by mastering change, thriving under pressure, and bouncing back from setbacks.

Wedemeyer, Richard, and Ronald Jue. *The Inner Edge: How to Integrate Your Life, Your Work, and Your Spirituality.* New York: McGraw-Hill 2004. Shows you how to make constructive and empowering changes by tapping into unknown resources of balance.

Yost, Cali. *Work + Life.* New York: The Berkeley Group, 2004. Provides a step-by-step plan to help you find practical answers to any unique work-life dilemma.

Support Organizations and Websites

Bryan E. Robinson, Ph.D.
www.bryanrobinsononline.com

A website with tips on how to outsmart stress, achieve work-life balance, and maintain stress resilience.

Workaholics Anonymous
www.workaholics-anonymous.org

World Service Organization
PO Box 289 Menlo Park, CA 94026-0289

A 12-Step support group that has chapters nationwide. Its purpose is to help people stop working compulsively.

INDEX

S

The Smart Guide Series

Making Smart People Smarter

THE SMART GUIDE TO

GREEN LIVING

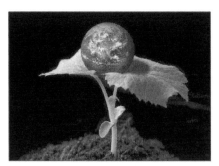

The most complete guide to green living ever published

How green living benefits your health as well as the Earth's

How green living can save you lots of money

Why the green economy and job market is an attractive, new, lucrative frontier

Julie Kerr **Gines**

Available Titles

Smart Guide To Astronomy
Smart Guide To Bachelorette Parties
Smart Guide To Back and Nerve Pain
Smart Guide To Biology
Smart Guide To Bridge
Smart Guide To Chemistry
Smart Guide To Classical Music
Smart Guide To Deciphering A Wine Label
Smart Guide To eBay
Smart Guide To Fighting Infections
Smart Guide To Forensic Careers
Smart Guide To Forensic Science
Smart Guide To Freshwater Fishing
Smart Guide To Getting Published
Smart Guide To Golf
Smart Guide To Green Living
Smart Guide To Healthy Grilling
Smart Guide To High School Math
Smart Guide To Hiking and Backpacking
Smart Guide To Horses and Riding
Smart Guide To Life After Divorce
Smart Guide To Making A Fortune With Infomercials
Smart Guide To Managing Stress
Smart Guide To Medical Imaging Tests
Smart Guide To Nutrition
Smart Guide To Patents
Smart Guide To Practical Math
Smart Guide To Single Malt Scotch
Smart Guide To Starting Your Own Business
Smart Guide To The Perfect Job Interview
Smart Guide To The Solar System
Smart Guide To Understanding Your Cat
Smart Guide To US Visas
Smart Guide To Wedding Weekend Events
Smart Guide To Wine

ABOUT THE AUTHOR

Bryan E. Robinson, Ph.D., is a psychotherapist, Professor Emeritus at the University of North Carolina at Charlotte, and a Fellow of the American Institute of Stress. He has authored thirty nonfiction books including *Chained to the Desk: A Guidebook for Workaholics, their Partners and Children, and the Clinicians who Treat Them, Don't Let Your Mind Stunt Your Growth*, and *Heal Your Self-Esteem*. His books have been translated into thirteen languages, and he has written for over one hundred professional journals and for such popular magazines as *Psychology Today, First for Women, American Health, Natural Health, Total Health, Lady's Circle, Complete Woman*, and *Psychotherapy Networker*. His column "Mindmatters" appeared monthly in *Your Health Magazine*. His work has been featured in *Town and Country, Marie Claire, McCall's, Mademoiselle, Out Magazine, Web MD, Shape, New Age Journal, Good Housekeeping, Men's Health, Women's Health, Ladies' Home Journal, Forbes, Fast Company, Fortune, Men's Journal, Best Life, The New York Times, Wall Street Journal, Chicago Tribune, Christian Science Monitor, The Atlanta Constitution, USA Today, New York Post*, and *The Miami Herald*.

He has won two awards for writing: the First Citizen's Scholars Medal from the University of North Carolina at Charlotte for excellence in scholarship, creativity, and/or research. The prestigious Extended Research Award from the American Counseling Association for his outstanding body of publications in the counseling field. He has lectured across the United States and throughout the world. His work has been featured on every major television network. He has appeared on ABC's *20/20, Good Morning America*, and ABC's *World News Tonight; NBC Nightly News, NBC Universal, the CBS Early Show, CNBC's The Big Idea*, and *CNN's Minding Your Money*, plus hundreds of local and national television and radio shows. He hosted the PBS documentary, *Overdoing It: When Work Rules Your Life*. He is a licensed psychotherapist with private practices in Charlotte and Asheville, NC. He resides in the Blue Ridge Mountains with his partner, four dogs and occasional bears at night. Visit his website at www.bryanrobinsononline.com or email him at bryanrobinson@bryanrobinsononline.com.